The Pediatric Airway

The Principles and Practice of the Pediatric Surgical Specialties

Edited by Stephen L. Gans, M.D.

Clinical Professor of Surgery
School of Medicine
University of California, Los Angeles
Attending in Surgery
Children's Hospital of Los Angeles
and Cedars-Sinai Medical Center
Los Angeles, California

This is the fourth book in the series.

H. BIEMANN OTHERSEN, JR., M.D.

Professor of Surgery and Pediatrics
Chief, Division of Pediatric Surgery
Medical University of South Carolina
Charleston, South Carolina

The
Pediatric
Airway

1991
W.B. SAUNDERS COMPANY
Harcourt Brace Jovanovich, Inc.
Philadelphia   London   Toronto   Montreal   Sydney   Tokyo

Megan Othersen, Research Editor

W. B. SAUNDERS COMPANY
Harcourt Brace Jovanovich, Inc.

The Curtis Center
Independence Square West
Philadelphia, PA 19106

Library of Congress Cataloging-in-Publication Data

The pediatric airway / edited by H. Biemann Othersen, Jr.
   p. cm. — (The Principles and practice of the pediatric
surgical specialties)
  ISBN 0-7216-2778-1
   1. Respiratory organs—Obstructions—Surgery.
  2. Respiratory organs—Abnormalities—Surgery.
  3. Children—Surgery.
  I. Othersen, H. Biemann. II. Series.
   [DNLM: 1. Airway Obstruction—in infancy & childhood.
WF 140 P371]
  RF51.P44 1991
  618.92′097533059—dc20
  DNLM/DLC   90-8868

Editor: Edward H. Wickland, Jr.

Developmental Editor: Kathleen McCullough

Designer: Ellen M. Bodner

Production Manager: Ken Neimeister

Manuscript Editor: Amy Eckenthal

Illustration Coordinator: Cecelia Kunkle

Indexer: Diana Witt

THE PEDIATRIC AIRWAY   ISBN   0-7216-2778-1

Printed in the United States of America

Last digit is the print number: 9 8 7 6 5 4 3 2 1

CONTRIBUTORS

NORMAN H. BRAHEN, M.D.
Assistant Professor of Anesthesiology and Director of Pediatric Anesthesiology, Medical University of South Carolina, Charleston, South Carolina
Anesthesia for the Child with Airway Problems

PAUL W. BRAUNSTEIN, JR., M.D.
Instructor in Surgery, Medical University of South Carolina, Charleston, South Carolina; Staff Surgeon, Virginia Beach General Hospital, Virginia Beach, Virginia
Vascular Malformations with Airway Obstruction

JOANNE M. CONROY, M.D.
Associate Professor of Anesthesiology, Medical University of South Carolina, Charleston, South Carolina
Anesthesia for the Child with Airway Problems

ROBIN T. COTTON, M.D.
Professor, University of Cincinnati College of Medicine; Director, Children's Hospital Medical Center, Cincinnati, Ohio

CATHERINE R. De VRIES, M.D.
Chief Resident, Urology, Department of Surgery, Stanford University School of Medicine, Stanford, California
Embryology and Development

PIETER A. De VRIES, M.D.
Clinical Professor of Surgery, Stanford University School of Medicine, Stanford, California; Chief of Pediatric Surgery, Santa Clara Valley Medical Center, San Jose, California
Embryology and Development

HOWARD EIGEN, M.D.
Professor of Pediatrics, Indiana University School of Medicine; Director, Section of Pediatric Pulmonology and Intensive Care, and Medical Director, Pediatric Intensive Care Unit, James Whitcomb Riley Hospital for Children, Indianapolis, Indiana
Pulmonary Physiology in the Surgical Infant

ROBERT M. FILLER, M.D.
Surgeon-in-Chief, Hospital for Sick Children, Toronto, Ontario, Canada
Tracheomalacia

STEPHEN L. GANS, M.D.
Clinical Professor of Surgery (Pediatric), UCLA School of Medicine; Chairman, Subdivision of Pediatric Surgery, Cedars-Sinai Medical Center, Los Angeles, California
Pediatric Endoscopy

JAY L. GROSFELD, M.D.
Lafayette F. Page Professor and Chairman, Department of Surgery, Indiana University School of Medicine; Surgeon-in-Chief, James Whitcomb Riley Hospital for Children, Indianapolis, Indiana
Pulmonary Physiology in the Surgical Infant

J. ALEX HALLER, JR., M.D.
Professor of Pediatric Surgery, Pediatrics, and Emergency Medicine, Johns Hopkins University School of Medicine; Children's Surgeon-in-Charge and Robert Garrett Professor of Pediatric Surgery, The Johns Hopkins Hospital, Baltimore, Maryland
Tracheostomy in Infants and Young Children

LUCINDA A. HALSTEAD, M.D.
Assistant Professor, Departments of Otolaryngology and Communicative Sciences and Pediatrics, Medical University of South Carolina; Consulting Physician, Veterans Administration Medical Center; Staff Physician, Charleston Memorial Hospital; Consulting Physician, St. Francis Xavier Hospital, Charleston, South Carolina
The Use of Lasers in the Pediatric Airway

DALE G. JOHNSON, M.D.
Professor of Surgery and Pediatrics, University of Utah School of Medicine; Surgeon-in-Chief, Primary Children's Medical Center; Head, Division of Pediatric Surgery, University of Utah Medical Center, Salt Lake City, Utah
Endoscopic Electrosurgical Resection of Subglottic Stenosis

ANN M. KOSLOSKE, M.D.
Clinical Professor of Surgery and Pediatrics, University of New Mexico School of Medicine; Director of Pediatric Surgery, The Children's Hospital of New Mexico, Albuquerque, New Mexico
Foreign Bodies in the Pediatric Airway

RODERICK I. MACPHERSON, M.D.
Professor, Radiology and Pediatrics, Medical University of South Carolina; Sec-

tion Head, Pediatric Radiology, Medical University of South Carolina Hospital, Charleston, South Carolina
Radiologic Aspects of Airway Obstruction

EUGENE D. McGAHREN, M.D.
Chief Resident, Department of Surgery, University of Virginia Health Sciences Center, Charlottesville, Virginia
Endotracheal Cryotherapy for Airway Strictures

HARRIET L. MAGRATH, R.N., M.S.N.
Pediatric Surgery Case Manager, Medical University of South Carolina Children's Hospital, Charleston, South Carolina
A Practical Guide to Home Care of the Child with a Tracheostomy

CHARLES M. MYER III, M.D.
Associate Professor, University of Cincinnati College of Medicine; Associate Professor, Children's Hospital Medical Center, Cincinnato, Ohio
Cricoid Split and Cartilage Tracheoplasty

H. BIEMANN OTHERSEN, JR., M.D.
Professor of Surgery and Pediatrics and Chief, Division of Pediatric Surgery, Medical University of South Carolina; Medical Director, Children's Hospital, Medical University of South Carolina Medical Center, Charleston, South Carolina
Medical Diseases of the Airway: A Surgeon's Role;
Subglottic Stenosis and Tracheobronchial Stricture: Classification and Therapy;
Tracheomalacia;
Injuries of the Airway: Extrinsic and Intrinsic;
Future Directions

BRADLEY M. RODGERS, M.D.
Professor of Surgery and Pediatrics, University of Virginia School of Medicine; Chief, Pediatric Surgery, University of Virginia Health Sciences Center, Charlottesville, Virginia
Endotracheal Cryotherapy for Airway Strictures

ROBERT M. SADE, M.D.
Professor of Cardiothoracic Surgery, Medical University of South Carolina; Chief of Pediatric Cardiac Surgery, Medical University of South Carolina Hospital, Charleston, South Carolina
Vascular Malformations with Airway Obstruction

C. D. SMITH, M.D.
Associate Professor of Surgery and Pediatrics, Medical University of South Carolina, Charleston, South Carolina
Subglottic Stenosis and Tracheobronchial Stricture: Classification and Therapy

CHARLES T. WALLACE, M.D.
Professor of Anesthesiology, Medical University of South Carolina; Director of Ambulatory Surgery, Medical University of South Carolina Hospital, Charleston, South Carolina
Anesthesia for the Child with Airway Problems

PREFACE

The origin of the medical sciences lies deeply entrenched in the realm of the arts. Historians have shown that medieval man was not without some knowledge of human anatomy; it was primarily philosophy, however, not physiology, upon which he relied when building his medical theories.

A belief surfaced during the Middle Ages in both China and India that illustrates the preponderance of philosophy in scientific theory. Eastern scholars postulated that the life principle, or the soul of man, resided in the body's respiratory passages. Medieval paintings that reflect this belief depict the soul as departing its earthly trappings by way of the mouth or nose, often in the form of a small bird (Fig. 1).

Although we no longer subscribe to such notions, the airway has managed to retain its medical significance. This is especially true in the case of the child; proper management of the pediatric airway is essential for the general health and well-being of every child. As illustrated in the philosophy of medieval China and by the treatment regimens presented in this book, the airway is nothing short of a primary concern. This is especially true in resuscitation. Correct management of the airway, often entailing only simple attention to details and an awareness of complications that may occur, will typically prevent a lifetime of problems.

The Pediatric Airway is a book intended for many specialists. The pediatric airway is the crossroads at which pediatricians, pediatric surgeons, otolaryngologists, thoracic surgeons, general surgeons, and plastic surgeons meet. The larynx, the trachea, and the bronchi, in some capacity, occupy each of these physicians' concern. Our interests in this book, however, are restricted; we will not be concerned with nasopharyngeal airway problems, such as choanal atresia or tonsillar hypertrophy, nor will we venture below the segmental bronchi. We will concentrate on the larynx, trachea, and main bronchi—these being, of course, the "seat of the soul."

This book is intended to present, in a straightforward manner, treatment regimens that have been found to be successful by a variety of specialists. Used exclusively throughout the book is a "how I do it" approach; the descriptions are intended to demonstrate treatment programs that have been found to be effective in the hands of well-trained and experienced pediatricians and sur-

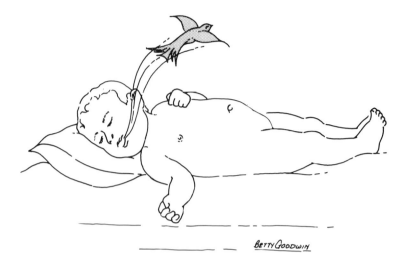

FIGURE 1

geons. These techniques are not, however, portrayed as the only effective treatment for the problem, and, in some cases, alternative methods of management
are presented as well. It must further be recognized that the simple, concise
presentation of technique is no indication that the procedure itself is simple or
easy and that any reader who follows the book's instructions can be assured of
success. There is no substitute for professional competence, extensive experience, and good training in the management of children and their airway
problems.

In the hands of well-trained, competent, and experienced pediatricians and
surgeons, this book should receive constant use. It is not intended to sit on the
shelf, deprived of all but the occasional reference.

When medical students are first introduced to the protocol for patient

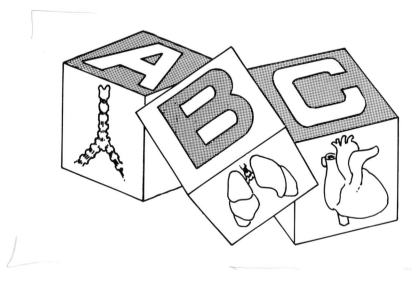

FIGURE 2

resuscitation, they are encouraged to use mnemonics in order to facilitate proper recall of the steps in the routine. They rememorize, in essence, their ABCs, the letter "A" referring to Airway, "B" to Breathing, and "C" to Circulation. I exhort my colleagues to refamiliarize themselves with their ABCs. In so doing, a thorough study of the pediatric airway is the place to begin (Fig. 2).

H. BIEMANN OTHERSEN, Jr., M.D.

FOREWORD

It's the Little Things That Count

As a pediatric surgeon, I have always maintained that "it's the little things that count." *The Pediatric Airway* examines the minute details, the seemingly small problems, that are often of great importance in the smallest people—children. In so doing, *The Pediatric Airway* provides the reader with an excellent discussion of congenital and acquired defects and diseases (including genesis, evaluation, differential diagnosis, and treatment) that seriously interfere with the normal respiration of infants and children.

In the early chapters, acknowledged authorities in the fields of embryology, physiology, and diagnostic radiology provide clear, easily understood background information, so necessary for precise clinical orientation toward a young patient with a major obstructive respiratory problem. This is followed by illustrated discussions of effective and preferred methods of management. The "what, how, and why" approach taken by the authors is refreshingly direct, easily digested, and oriented toward results. In simple language, each writer details *what* he or she is going to do, *how* he or she is going to do it, and, finally, *why* that approach was chosen.

A discussion of tracheostomy in infants and children winds things up. The selection of equipment, the technical procedure, and the management of a child with a tracheostomy (with or without respiratory support, in the hospital and the home) are covered in detail.

I envision *The Pediatric Airway* as a well-worn, dog-eared single reference book, handily available to and used by many: anesthesiologists, surgical specialists, pediatricians, and nursing personnel—all those big people who care for the increasing number of infants and young children requiring acute or long-term evaluation of congenital, iatrogenic, or otherwise acquired major obstructive lesions of the laryngotracheobronchial tree.

To repeat: It's the little things—the little books and the little people—that count.

H. WILLIAM CLATWORTHY, JR., M.D.
Emeritus Professor of Surgery
Ohio State University
Columbus, Ohio

CONTENTS

part **5**
Future Directions

part 1

General Considerations in Infants and Children

chapter 1

Embryology and Development

Pieter A. De Vries, M.D.
Catherine R. De Vries, M.D.

This chapter focuses on the embryology and subsequent development of the larynx, trachea, and bronchi. To understand the normal and pathologic development of the airway, it is necessary to comprehend the contributions of their primordial tissues. Materials included our own collection of staged, serially sectioned embryos and, through the courtesy of Professor Dr. Ronan O'Rahilly, the collection of human embryos and fetuses at the Carnegie Laboratories of Embryology in Davis, California.

The "embryonic" period of human development is confined to the first 8 weeks after conception. During this time, the zygote (fertilized oocyte) evolves into an embryo of about 30 mm in length and 2 to 2.7 gm in weight. Each of the 23 embryonic stages of development is defined by morphologic characteristics rather than size or chronologic age. The "fetal" period encompasses the remainder of prenatal life and is not divided into recognized stages.

Early Morphogenesis

During the second embryonic stage, successive cellular divisions lead to the formation of a 16-cell embryo called a *morula*. The fate of each of these cells is believed to be determined by topographic position. Peripheral cells become the extraembryonic trophectoderm (trophoblast). The inner cell mass (ICM), however, is the root of all of the intraembryonic and the remainder of the extraembryonic formative tissues (Fig. 1–1A). The third embryonic stage (ovulation age of 4 days) is called a *blastocyst* and derives its name from the fluid-filled cavity that develops within the trophectoderm beneath the polarly placed ICM

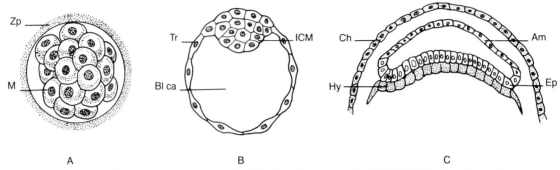

A   B   C

FIGURE 1-1. *A,* Stage 2 embryo. Note the morula *(M)* within the zona pellucida *(Zp). B,* Section of stage 3 embryo, a blastocyst. Outer cells of morula have become trophectoderm *(Tr),* whereas inner cells have become inner cell mass *(ICM). Bl ca,* blastocyst cavity. *C,* Section of stage 5c embryo, a bilaminar embryonic disc. *Ch,* chorion; *Am,* amnion; *Ep,* epiblast; *Hy,* hypoblast.

(Fig. 1–1*B*). Over the next week (stages 4 and 5), the blastocyst attaches to and becomes implanted in the uterine wall. During this period, some cells *(blastomeres)* of the ICM form a plate, adjacent to the polar trophoblast, called the *epiblast* (primary ectoderm). Other cells of the ICM delaminate to form, below the epiblast, a plate called the *hypoblast* (primitive or primary endoderm). Together, the epiblast and the hypoblast constitute the bilaminar *embryonic disc.* A proliferation of cells from the edges of the epiblast form the overlying amnion and amniotic cavity (Fig. 1–1*C*).

The hypoblast was formerly believed to be the root of the endodermal epithelium. It has now been shown, however, that the hypoblast does not contribute to the embryonic gut or its derivatives but is restricted to the extraembryonic epithelium of the umbilical stalk and the lining of the umbilical vesicle (vitelline or yolk sac).

The cells of the gut endoderm and the embryonic mesoblast originate in the epiblast. By about 2 weeks of age (stage 6), the epiblast has become an epithelial layer with typical cellular gap junctions and a basal lamina. It can be viewed as a "mosaic" with areas designated to form specific tissues of specific organs. The process by which the "presumptive" gut endoderm cells and "presumptive" mesoblast cells move from their specific areas of the epiblast into the hypoblast is called *gastrulation.*

Migration of Cells

In human embryos, by the end of the 2nd week (stage 6b) there is an acceleration of cellular proliferation and a caudomedial movement of cells of the epiblast (Fig. 1–2*A*). As they converge, a loss of basal lamina and tight cell junctions result in the piling up of cells and the formation of the primitive node and primitive streak (Fig. 1–2*B*). Those cells at the node and streak invaginate and detach from the epiblast. Those of the presumptive gut endoderm, including the prerespiratory epithelium, colonize the underlying hypoblastic layer of loosely associated cells. Cells of the presumptive mesoblast migrate laterally and rostrally between the epiblast and hypoblast.

The following facts regarding the lung's epiblastic sites of origin and their

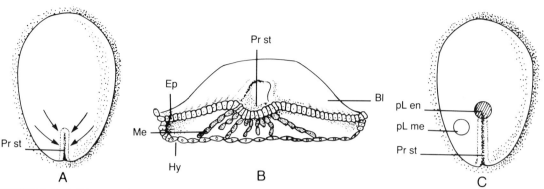

FIGURE 1-2. *A,* Diagram of caudomedial movements of epiblast cells toward the evolving primitive streak *(Pr st). B,* Transverse section through embryo at the level of the primitive streak. *Ep,* epiblast; *Me,* mesoblast; *Hy,* hypoblast; *Bl,* basal lamina. *C,* Areas of the epiblast in medium-streak chick (stage 6b human) determined to become prelung endoderm *(pL en)* and prelung mesoblast *(pL me).* (Redrawn from Rosenquist GC: The origin and movement of prelung cells in the chick embryo as determined by radio autographic mapping. J Embryol Exp Morph 24:497–509, 1970.)

cellular migration paths have been abstracted from experimental studies on chick embryos.[14]

"Medium-streak" stage (late stage 6). The presumptive endodermal cells that form the prerespiratory epithelium of the "lung" reside within the rostral (cranial) third of the primitive streak, whereas the prelung mesoblast is located halfway between the lateral edge of the epiblast and the streak (Fig. 1–2C). The prelung mesoblast participates in the centripetal movement of epiblast cells toward the elongating primitive streak.

"Definitive-streak" stage. The endodermal cells have left the streak but remain in the region, implanted in the hypoblast. The mesoblast has begun its migration through the streak.

"Head-process" stage (human stage 7, or 16 days). The prelung endoderm has migrated "away from the streak into the zone of endoderm destined for the ventrolateral wall of the gut." Concomitantly the prelung mesoderm has "migrated from the streak into the mesoderm destined for the part of the lateral plate between the kidney and the heart-forming region."

Two- to three-somite stage. The foregut begins as a dorsal outpouching near the cranial end of the endoderm. The prelung endoderm lies lateral and caudal (Fig. 1–3A).

Nine- to ten-somite stage in chicks (human stage 10). The prelung endoderm is partially folded into the foregut (Fig. 1–3B and C). In the human (stage 11), the prelung mesoblast has "migrated" into the splanchnic mesoblast and then becomes more closely adherent "to the ventral wall of the gut" (Fig. 1–3D).

Rosenquist concluded from these observations of the chick that the two lung precursors, the endoderm and mesoderm, migrate separately and do not come into "intimate contact" in the chick until the 16- to 19-somite stage.

It is quite reasonable to assume that the same development occurs in humans. In the 18-somite human embryo (stage 11) the laryngotracheopulmonary primordium occupies the ventral and ventrolateral walls of the foregut. This "respiratory groove" is just above the hepatic diverticulum. It has tall columnar epithelium, which becomes multilayered, especially caudally. At that point the respiratory diverticulum can be seen as an evolving ventral expansion of the groove in the 28-somite embryos. However, even before this epithelial bulge

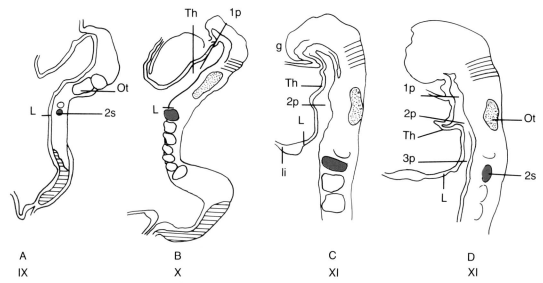

FIGURE 1–3. Median sections through four embryos, redrawn and modified from Bartelmez and Evans (1926). *A*, Stage 9, 2-somite embryo. *B*, Stage 10, 8-somite embryo. *C*, Stage 11, 11-somite embryo. *D*, Stage 11, 16-somite embryo. *Ot*, optic disc; *2s*, second somite; *Th*, thyroid primordium; *li*, liver. *1p*, *2p*, and *3p* are areas of the first, second, and third pharyngeal pouches as they arise and develop from the foregut endoderm. *L* shows the rostroventral migration of the pulmonary primordium.

appears, the site of this diverticulum can be identified in 25-somite embryos by the protrusion of the visceral mesodermal wall into the coelom. There is no doubt that the epithelial and mesodermal primordia of the larynx, trachea, and primary bronchi are, at that stage, located in juxtaposition in the ventral wall of the foregut. Individual boundaries between the trachea, larynx, and bronchi cannot be defined (Fig. 1–4).

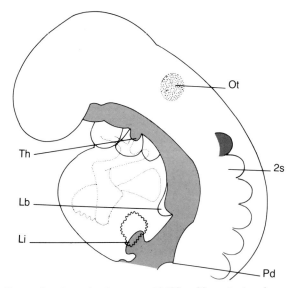

FIGURE 1–4. A median section through a late stage 12 (28 to 29 somites) embryo with developing lung bud *(Lb)*. Large arrows demarcate the rostrocaudal limits of the ventral laryngotracheopulmonary area of the foregut (stippled) epithelium. Other midline foregut "buds" shown are *Th*, thyroid; *Li*, liver; and *Pd*, dorsal pancreas. *Ot*, otic disc; *2s*; second somite. Heart and arterial arches are shown in dotted lines.

BRONCHI

By the end of the 4th week (stages 12 and 13), a singular "lung bud" appears. Shortly thereafter, right and left lung buds (primary bronchi) are evident even before the trachea is recognizable. The left bud grows transversely, whereas the right bud becomes slightly longer and is directed caudally.

The outgrowth of the lung bud's endodermal epithelium is induced by the surrounding pulmogenic mesoderm. To develop further branching,[16] the pulmonic mesoblast of the pulmonary coelum into which the lung buds bulge is necessary (Fig. 1–5).

During the 5th week (stages 14 and 15), mesenchymal proliferation ceases and the thinned epithelium of the pulmonary coelomic wall becomes the visceral pleura. The pulmonary primordium grows caudally and laterally as the trachea and esophagus evolve and lengthen. The tracheobronchial junction (carina) then lies in front of the esophagus with the bronchi laterally. Three lobar buds appear on the right and two on the left (Fig. 1–6A). Capillary plexuses surround the condensing mesenchyme, a pulmonary vein enters the left atrium, and plexiform pulmonary arteries will develop into the pulmonary circulation.

In the 6th week (stages 16 and 17) with continued growth, the primary bronchi straddle the esophagus. The lobar bronchi lengthen, and by the end of this period all the segmental buds have appeared (Fig. 1–6B).

During the 7th week (stages 18 and 19), further divisions of subsegmental bronchi appear, and by the end of this week the lungs fill only half of the pleural cavities (which are not yet separated from the peritoneal cavity). The arborization of the lungs' larger airway passages is complete with the larger bronchi lined by pseudostratified ciliated epithelium.

Formation of new small bronchi continues through the 16th week, and

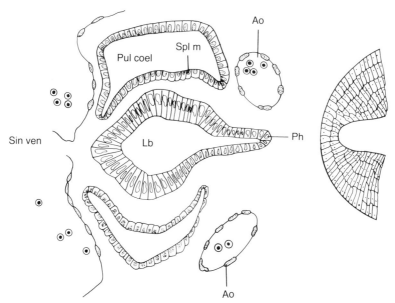

FIGURE 1–5. Transverse section of a late stage 12 embryo showing lung bud *(Lb)* bulging into the pulmonary coelom *(pul coel)*. The "epithelium" of the medial wall of the cavity, the splanchnic mesoblast *(Spl m)*, is a proliferative source of pulmonary mesoblast. *Sin ven,* sinus venosus; *Ph,* pharynx; *Ao,* right and left aortae.

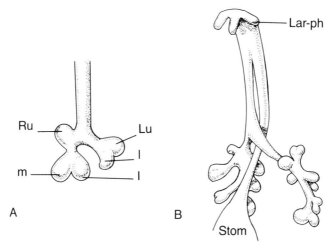

FIGURE 1–6. *A,* Epithelium of lobar buds (late stage 14). *Ru,* right upper; *m,* middle; *Lu,* left upper; and *l,* lower lobe buds. *B,* Segmental buds (stage 17). *Lar-ph,* laryngopharynx; *Stom,* stomach.

smaller air passages are formed for nearly a decade into postnatal life. Cartilage formation, which starts around 10 weeks in the primary bronchi, continues to appear through 24 weeks.

TRACHEA

In primitive fish the trachea appears as a single ventral pharyngeal diverticulum with paired lungs even before a primitive larynx is noted in amphibians. The best evidence suggests that the trachea arises in mammals as part of the "lung bud," at the caudal end of the pharyngeal "respiratory groove."

Until recently, it was generally believed that the separation of the trachea from the esophagus was the result of an active ascending division of a common tracheoesophageal primordium. This division was thought to occur by the upward intrusion of a mesenchymal wedge into the notch between the lung bud and the foregut followed by fusion of the lateral foregut wall.[6] Later, Smith[15] proposed that fusion of lateral epithelial ridges, within the foregut, divided a common tracheoesophageal primordium. Necrosis of cells at the tracheoesophageal junction was thought to be followed by passive "filling in" of mesoblast to form a "tracheoesophageal septum."[15]

Zaw-Tun[24] disagreed and denied the existence of a "tracheoesophageal septum." He felt that the ventrally arching caudal wall of the lung bud's neck was the "primitive pharyngeal floor" and that the foregut cavity immediately above it was the "primitive pharynx." He stated, "The respiratory primordium is drawn cranialward; it proliferates, dilates, bifurcates, and grows caudally, dragging out a stalk from the ventral aspect of the foregut. Most of the stalk above the bifurcation will develop into the trachea." He felt that the cranial portion of the "stalk" became the glottis and infraglottic portion of the larynx.

It is highly unlikely that a "stalk" is merely "drawn out" respiratory epithelium, although the larynx, trachea, and lungs do develop from adjacent regions of the ventral wall. Wessels described in the mouse an inductive tracheogenic mesoderm that inhibits the formation of bronchial buds, whereas bronchiogenic mesoderm evokes the formation of bronchial buds.[23]

O'Rahilly and Muller[12] describe the tracheoesophageal septum as the mesoblast between the dorsal epithelial wall of the trachea and the ventral wall of the esophagus. They also felt that, during most of the embryonic period, the apex of the tracheoesophageal segment remained at a constant level. They found that the growth in length of the esophagus exceeds that of the trachea.

Zaw-Tun's "primitive pharyngeal floor" implies that the lung, trachea, and infraglottic larynx are derivatives of the pharynx. This theory is likely but arguable. During stages 12 and 13, the wall of the evolving lung bud must contain, or at least be surrounded by, different primordia at different time intervals, i.e., first pulmogenic, then tracheogenic, and finally laryngogenic. Thus the cranial mesoblast separating the epithelium of the foregut from that of the lung bud cannot be correctly viewed as a tracheoesophageal septum during these stages. Later, in stage 14, the area of mesoblast separating the epithelial stalk, above the primary bronchial buds, from the ventral foregut wall might be considered a "tracheoesophageal septum" if one considers the infraglottic portion of the larynx as part of the trachea. These uncertainties leave the "separation point" undefined.

By stage 15 (about 33 days), the mesoblast around the trachea and esophagus shows signs of separation. The cells become oriented in a lamellar fashion around each epithelial tube, and each mesoblastic coat is surrounded by a capillary plexus. The vagus nerves are seen laterally, just outside the individual coats, but within a more peripheral, common coat.

Progressive differentiation of the tracheal and esophageal walls during the next three stages results in their marked dissimilarity in stage 18 (7th week) (Fig. 1–7). The trachea has a dense, precartilaginous coat, whereas the esophagus has a thick submucosal layer and surrounding muscular coats. Cartilage appears in the trachea in stage 20.

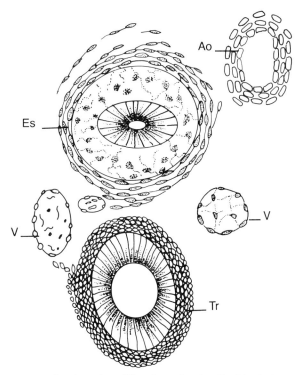

FIGURE 1-7. Transverse section in a stage 17 embryo showing the histologic appearances of the trachea *(Tr)* and esophagus *(Es)*. *V,* vagus nerves; *Ao,* aorta. The trachea has a thick connective tissue, i.e., precartilaginous layer around the epithelium, whereas the esophagus has a premuscular coat around a thick submucosa.

LARYNX

The larynx is first seen in amphibians as a slitlike glottis bounded by a pair of lateral cartilages. In reptiles the forerunner of the epiglottis can be seen cranial to the glottis, but a thyroid cartilage is not seen prior to crocodilians. The mammalian larynx thus can be thought of as consisting of two parts: the more ancient, the infraglottic part, is related primarily to ventilation, and the more recent, the supraglottic, is associated with the development of vocal function.

Anatomically the larynx is a composite structure. The supraglottic part uses the hyoid bone for support and is supplied by the superior laryngeal nerves and arteries. Its lymphatics drain to the deep cervical nodes. The glottic and infraglottic structures (true vocal cords and below) are supplied by the recurrent nerves and the inferior laryngeal arteries and nerves. Lymphatics from this area drain to the pre- and peritracheal nodes.

Laryngeal Cavities

The development of the human larynx reflects the larynx's phylogenetic history. The infraglottic cavity develops first, followed much later by the vestibule and, even later, the ventricle of the supraglottic cavity. Finally, the vocal cords appear.

The infraglottic cavity is above and continuous with the trachea and may be considered a part of the trachea. It appears to arise as a conical part of the cranial end of the elongating respiratory diverticulum in stages 13 and 14. A narrowed infraglottic space in stage 15 has been called the "pharyngotracheal duct" (Fig. 1–8A). By stage 16, the duct has become so narrowed, perhaps by

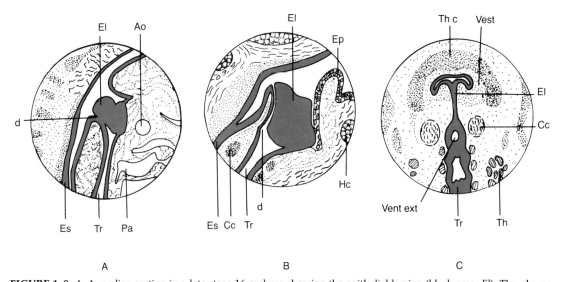

A   B   C

FIGURE 1-8. *A*, A median section in a late stage 16 embryo showing the epithelial lamina (black area, *El*). The pharyngotracheal duct *(d)* is most narrow dorsorostrally. *Ao*, aorta; *Pa*, pulmonary artery (trunk); *Es*, esophagus; *Tr*, trachea. *B*, Stage 19 embryo with the same plane of section and magnification as in Figure 1–8A. Note the elongation of the pharyngotracheal duct *(d)*. *Ep*, epiglottis; *Cc*, cricoid precartilage; *Hc*, cartilaginous hyoid bone. *C*, Coronal section at same magnification and embryonic stage as in Figure 1–8B. It shows the ventral extension *(Vent ext)* of the "cricoid duct" portion of the infraglottic cavity. It is flanked by the cricoid precartilage *(Cc)*. Dorsal to the thyroid cartilage *(Th c)* is the coronal cleft of the vestibule *(Vest)*. The sagittal primordia of the vestibule, the epithelial lamina *(El)*, extends dorsocaudally. Portions of the thyroid gland *(Th)* can be seen lateral to the tracheal precartilage.

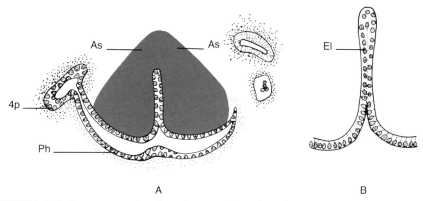

FIGURE 1-9. *A,* Transverse section through a stage 15 embryo showing the ''arytenoid swellings'' *(As),* condensations of mesoblast adjoining the median epithelial lamina, laryngeal groove, and pharynx *(Ph). B,* Orderly single layer of cuboidal cells of the laryngeal groove extends ventrally as the pectiniform epithelial lamina *(El).*

stretching, that its lumen often appears obliterated. Subsequently the infraglottic cavity enlarges caudally as the surrounding cricoid cartilage acquires a circular form in stages 19 and 20 (Fig. 1–8*B*). Cranially the enlargement is due to the formation of the ''subglottic recess,'' first described by Walander in the rat.[19] It is an extension of the infraglottic cavity into the bulbous portion of the epithelial lamina and is probably brought about by cell necrosis (Fig. 1–8*C*).

The supraglottic cavity evolves by a rather complicated interrelationship between the respiratory epithelium of the laryngeal groove and lateral masses of mesoblast, the arytenoid swellings, derived from the sixth visceral arch (Fig. 1–9*A*). The laryngeal groove consists of the converging ventral and lateral walls of the foregut, from the lowest pharyngeal pouch to the lung bud. It has generally been believed that the ventral projection of this laryngeal groove, the ''epithelial lamina,'' which extends from the top of the groove to the level of the pharyngotracheal duct, is formed by an ''epithelial fusion'' of the walls of the groove caused by their median compression from the expanding, lateral arytenoid swellings. However, Walander showed in rats that the epithelial lamina arose as a solid ventral outgrowth from the laryngeal groove, rather than from an epithelial fusion of the lateral walls.[19]

This pectiniform outgrowth can first be seen in both rat and man in stage 13, prior to the emergence of distinctive arytenoid swellings. However, in human embryos in stages 13 through 16, the epithelial lamina consists of two adjoining parts: the dorsal part, extending from the epithelial walls of the laryngeal groove, and the ventral part, which is more solid and appears to be identical to that seen in the rat (Fig. 1–9*B*).

Muller and colleagues[9] have suggested that after fusion of right and left epithelial layers to form a lamina, there is a proliferation of cells during which time they become irregularly arranged. Then, at the end of the embryonic period the cells rearrange and separation takes place. Study of a large number of specially stained sections of human embryos in stages 12 through 15 will likely be required to further clarify the manner in which the epithelial lamina forms. The development of the larynx is dependent on the lamina's initial formation, proliferation, and sequential cavitations.

At the cranial end of the epithelial lamina, there are bilateral budding outgrowths in stage 16 (about 37 days). Each lateral bud forms a lumen with fusion

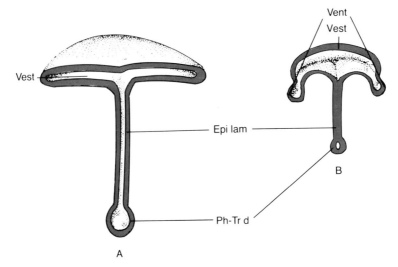

FIGURE 1-10. *A,* The coronal sulcus of the vestibule *(Vest),* which tapers ventrocaudally. The epithelial lamina *(Epi lam)* extends dorsally and terminates at the pharyngotracheal duct *(Ph-Tr d). B,* At the caudolateral part of the coronal vestibule *(Vest),* solid ventricle buds develop lumens *(Vent)* toward the end of the embryonic period of development.

medially to form a coronal cavity. This cavity becomes the vestibule, which is the primary supraglottic cavity (Fig. 1–10*A*). By the beginning of the 8th week (stages 19 and 20), the primordia of the ventricles begin to form. These additions to the supraglottic cavity originate in solid budlike outgrowths from the epithelial walls of the vestibular cavity. The ventricular buds develop lumens that communicate with the vestibule (Fig. 1–10*B*).

By the end of the 8th week (stage 23, or the last of the embryonic stages), dissolution of the epithelial lamina has begun. When this occurs, the vestibular cavity is enlarged, but the glottic aperture does not appear until about 10 weeks (40 mm). At that time, a central dissolution of the epithelial lamina occurs in the area between supraglottic and infraglottic chambers. The ventricles then constitute a "middle compartment" of the larynx, between the vestibular folds (false cords) and vocal cords (true cords) (Fig. 1–11*A*).

Cartilages and Muscles

The thyroid, cricoid, and epiglottic cartilages are first recognizable in the 7th week (stage 18) as condensations of mesenchyme (precartilage). The arytenoids are the last of the major cartilages to appear, and by stage 21 all but the epiglottic cartilage have undergone development into their mature configurations.

The development of the cricoid during this period is of particular interest because of its relationship with the subglottic lumen. Subglottic stenosis may be of congenital etiology and follows in frequency only laryngomalacia and vocal cord paralysis among congenital laryngeal anomalies. The congenital subglottic stenosis may be either a generalized circumferential narrowing at the cricoid lumen or an abnormal shape of the cartilage.

In embryos of stage 18, the mesenchyme condenses most markedly ventrally, thins laterally, and then thickens again dorsally. The lumen is slitlike, and the sides appear compressed. The cricoid expands very rapidly to become a com-

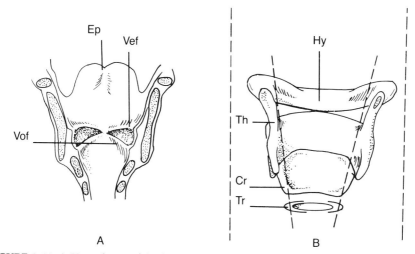

FIGURE 1–11. *A*, Ventral area of the larynx in the neonate viewed from behind. The ventricle, or "third cavity," is bounded from above by the ventricular folds *(Vef)* and from below by the vocal folds *(Vof)*. *Ep*, epiglottis. *B*, Laryngeal cartilages (without arytenoids). *Th*, thyroid; *Cr*, cricoid; *Tr*, trachea; and *Hy*, hyoid viewed from behind. Inner dotted line shows telescopic configuration in the neonate as opposed to the rectangular shape in the adult (outer dotted line).

plete ring, whereas the lumen enlarges and becomes circular in shape. In its final normal configuration the cricoid has a much more extensive dorsal than ventral lamina.

The premuscle masses appear at the same time as the precartilage. By the end of the 7th week (stage 19), the muscles are well differentiated, have developed striations, and are innervated.

RELATIONSHIPS OF RESPIRATORY STRUCTURES

It has been thought that during the 4th through the 6th weeks of embryonic life the pharyngotracheal duct orifice shifts cranially relative to the cervical ganglia and vertebrae. The separation point of trachea and esophagus has appeared to some investigators to remain at a stable level. Thereafter their relative positions remain constant until the latter part of the fetal period, when a caudal shift begins and continues after birth. Descent of the larynx is most marked during the first 2 years but continues until about 6 years of age.

At birth the larynx of a term fetus is small compared with the mouth and pharynx, although there is considerable variation in normal laryngeal size. The epiglottis of the newborn is short and small, and the valleculae are shallow so that the tongue approximates the epiglottis. The larynx points toward the nasopharynx, thus facilitating nasal breathing. The arytenoid apparatus is large in proportion to the lumen of the larynx. In the newborn the subglottic region is narrower than the glottic aperture. Each successive cartilage, from cranial to caudal (hyoid to cricoid), telescopically fits within the one above (Fig. 1–11*B*). In the adult configuration, the glottic aperture, not the cricoid, is the narrowest point of the airway lumen.

Growth of the larynx and epiglottis is rapid for the first 3 years after birth, and then growth slows. By 3 years of age the epiglottis has developed its adult configuration. The various dimensions of the larynx have been shown to have a linear relationship, not to age, but to the crown-heel length of the individual. At puberty there is another growth spurt, particularly in males.[2]

ANOMALIES OF THE AIRWAY

Bronchi

Anomalies in the patterns of lobes, segments, and subsegments are the result of variations in the site at which respective buds arise. These anomalies are usually not significant unless they are associated with abnormal function or predispose the individual to disease, e.g., a precarinal right upper lobe orifice or a pulmonary sequestration.

Smith[15] felt that "accessory" and "sequestered" lobes should be distinguished, as he believed the former arose earlier in development. However, their similarities in development indicate that they are both sequestrations, one lobar ("accessory") and the other segmental. Both, as a rule, derive their arterial blood supply from the aorta rather than from a pulmonary artery. Usually, neither lobar nor segmental sequestrations have patent bronchial communications with the remainder of the lung. Both usually involve the left lower lobe. Lobar buds do appear in stage 15 about 1 week before segmental buds appear in stage 17. This could account for the difference in venous return in that the venous drainage of segmental sequestrations is to pulmonary veins, whereas the lobar sequestrations usually drain to extrapulmonary veins, such as the azygous. However, a right lower lobe sequestration has been found with venous return to the portal circulation. The capillary plexuses surrounding the "lung" and lobar buds are initially related to the "systemic" circulation. The pulmonary venous channels to the single pulmonary vein are established at a relatively early age, but they do not accompany the evolving bronchi as arborization takes place.

However, the outgrowth of the buds is normally associated with a similar extension of the elongating pulmonary arteries. Whatever causes the loss of continuity of the lobar or segmental bud from the remainder of the lung obviously does the same to the accompanying pulmonary artery. The primary arterial channels of the lobe or segment arise from the aorta.

Trachea

Esophageal atresia with a fistula between the trachea and the distal esophageal segment is the most common anomaly of the suprapulmonary defects. Many hypotheses have been put forth to explain these developments. In 1957, Smith[15] ascribed the tracheoesophageal defects to the faulty union of the internal epithelial ridges. However, Zaw-Tun[24] evaluated the same and similar embryonic material and disagreed.

O'Rahilly and Muller[12] attributed the spectrum of tracheoesophageal anomalies to a secondary tracheoesophageal union and esophageal disruption in stage 15. At this stage, the carina straddles the ventral wall of the elongating esophagus. Arguments against a secondary tracheoesophageal fistula, with or without an esophageal atresia, during stage 15 include the following: (1) a significant number of tracheoesophageal fistulae with esophageal atresia arise proximal to the carina; (2) tracheoesophageal fistulae without esophageal atresia are usually located even more cranially; and (3) in stage 15, the trachea and esophagus have developed dissimilar surrounding mesoblastic coats, which would appear to make a secondary epithelial union unlikely.

Considering current views on the mechanisms of pathogenesis, it appears to us that tracheoesophageal anomalies can be related to one of two possible mechanisms. First, there could be an aberrant location and/or quantity of their primordia by stage 13. To avoid structural abnormality, appropriate numbers of properly determined cells within a genetically normal epiblast must have made their way to the proper place in the developing foregut. Any interference with such cellular replications and morphogenetic movements would result in such an anomaly. Second, a general metabolic disturbance during stage 13 could adversely affect cell proliferation and interactions.

Following observations of the sequential development of the foregut, one cannot escape the conclusion that during stages 12 and 13 a circumferential area of the foregut wall shares the primordia of the infraglottic part of the larynx, the trachea, the lower pharynx, and a portion of the esophagus dorsally. There are no markers for the pharyngoesophageal junction. However, in rat embryos, the ventral respiratory epithelium can be distinguished from the dorsal epithelium of the prepharynx and preesophagus. In the region of the foregut under consideration here, the presumptive laryngotracheal epithelium occupies the largest part of the circumference, all but the small dorsal wall.

With the foregoing observations, one might imagine different explanations of tracheoesophageal anomalies. One explanation is as follows: If the mesenchymal tracheogenic primordium, surrounding a part of the respiratory epithelium, were to extend further dorsally into the presumptive esophageal area, theoretically it could interrupt the esophagus and still maintain a communication between the trachea and esophagus distally. A delay in the normal migration of this tracheogenic mesoblast could provide the hypothetical mechanism.

All of these theories should be viewed at this time as pure speculation. The lack of precise morphometric data for a convincing description of normal development in the early embryonic stages warrants no more.

Larynx

The most common gross morphologic anomaly, subglottic stenosis involving the cricoid cartilage, has been discussed previously. The next most common partial obstruction is caused by a web formation at the anterior commissure. The dorsal extension of the web usually involves two thirds of the vocal cords and may be up to 1 cm in thickness. Membranes consist of mesodermal derivatives (muscle and connective tissue), epithelium, and glands. Walander[20] attributed this defect to a partial failure in the formation of the subglottic recess.

Most atresias of the larynx involve a failure of formation of the subglottic recess.

Supraglottic and infraglottic or "total" atresia can be ascribed to the failure of vestibular outgrowth and subglottic recess formation. What develops is a supraglottic cavity that is filled by a muscle mass and approximated arytenoid cartilages with midline fusion. The infraglottic cavity is replaced by a malformed cricoid mass. However, the pharyngotracheal duct persists, as it does in all forms of laryngeal "atresia."

Walander believed these malformations to be "fundamentally due to premature arrest of the normally vigorous epithelial activity." His theoretical views are consistent with observed development in the rat, and no more plausible theory has been found. Little or nothing is known of epithelial-mesenchymal interactions during development in this region.

Further conjecture concerning laryngeal defects should await a clarification of normal developmental relationships of the larynx, trachea, and esophagus.

REFERENCES

1. Bellairs R: The primitive streak. Anat Embryol 174:1–4, 1986
2. Bosma JF: Anatomy of the Infant Head. Baltimore, The Johns Hopkins University Press, 1986
3. Boyden EA: Notes on the development of the lung in infancy and childhood. Am J Anat 121:749–762, 1967
4. Frazer E: Development of the larynx. J Anat Physiol 44:156–191, 1910
5. Gardner RL: Regeneration of endoderm from the ectoderm in the mouse embryo: Fact or artifact? J Embryol Exp Morph 88:303–326, 1985
6. His W: Anatomie menschlicher Embryonen. III. Zur Geschichte der Organe. Leipzig, Vogel, 1885, pp 12–19
7. Lisser H: Studies in the development of the human larynx. Am J Anat 12:26–66, 1911
8. Luckett WP: Origin and differentiation of the yolk sac and extra-embryonic mesoderm in human embryos and Rhesus monkey embryos. Am J Anat 152:59–98, 1978
9. Muller F, O'Rahilly R, Tucker JA: The human larynx at the end of the embryonic period proper. Ann Otol Rhinol Laryngol 94:607–617, 1985
10. O'Rahilly R, Boyden EA: The timing and sequence of events in the development of the human respiratory system during the embryonic period. Z Anat Entwickl-G Esch 141:237–250, 1973
11. O'Rahilly R, Muller F: Developmental stages in human embryos. Contrib Embryol Carnegie Inst Wash, 637:1–306, 1987
12. O'Rahilly R, Muller F: Respiratory and alimentary relations in staged human embryos. Ann Otol Rhinol Laryngol 93:421–429, 1984
13. Poelman RE: The head-process and the formation of the definitive endoderm in the mouse embryo. Anat Embryol 162:41–49, 1981
14. Rosenquist GC: The origin and movement of prelung cells in the chick embryo as determined by radio autographic mapping. J Embryol Exp Morph 23:497–509, 1970
15. Smith EI: The early development of the trachea and esophagus in relation to atresia of the esophagus and tracheoesophageal fistula. Contrib Embryol Carnegie Inst Wash 31:27–63, 1957
16. Spooner BS, Wessels NK: Mammalian lung development: Interactions in primordium formation and bronchial morphogenesis. J Exp Zool 175:445–454, 1970
17. Streeter GL: Developmental horizons in human embryos. Description of age groups XV, XVI, XVII, XVIII, being the third issue of a survey of the Carnegie Collection. Contrib Embryol Carnegie Inst Wash, 32:133–203, 1948
18. Tucker JA, O'Rahilly R: Observations on the embryology of the human larynx. Ann Otol 81:520–523, 1972
19. Walander A: Prenatal development of the epithelial primordium of the larynx in rat. Acta Anat 10 (Suppl 13):1–140, 1950
20. Walander A: The mechanism of origin of congenital malformations of the larynxol. Acta Otolaryngol 45:426–432, 1955
21. Wells LJ: Development of the human diaphragm and pleural sacs. Contrib Embryol Carnegie Inst Wash 35:107–134, 1954
22. Wells LJ, Boyden EA: The development of bronchopulmonary segments in human embryos of horizons XVII to XIX. Am J Anat 95:163–201, 1954
23. Wessels NK: Mammalian lung development: Interactions in formation and morphogenesis of tracheal buds. J Exp Zool 175:455–466, 1970
24. Zaw-Tun HA: The tracheo-esophageal septum—fact or fantasy? Acta Anat 114:1–21, 1982

chapter 2

Pulmonary Physiology in the Surgical Infant

Howard Eigen, M.D.
Jay L. Grosfeld, M.D.

It hardly needs to be stated that the infant is very different from the adult; this may be especially true and often least recognized in regard to the respiratory system.

The infant labors under several respiratory disadvantages:

1. An infant's airways are narrow and therefore may easily become obstructed, and collateral ventilation is poorly developed.
2. Whereas the infant's chest wall is more compliant than that of the adult, the lungs are less compliant, a factor that results in low functional residual capacity (FRC).
3. The infant's respiratory muscles fatigue easily and cannot compensate well for stress placed on the respiratory system by disease.

The healthy infant normally lives on the edge of respiratory failure with less reserve than older children and adults; the disruption of his or her milieu by illness or an operation can easily result in respiratory difficulty. The more immature the infant, the fewer respiratory units and the less surface area available for adequate ventilation.

RESPIRATORY SYSTEM MECHANICS

The recoil of the chest wall is zero in the mature fetus.[1,2] Although there is a progressive increase in outward recoil as the child matures (Fig. 2–1), chest wall compliance remains very high in infants compared with the same value in older children and adults.

The compliance of the chest wall in the newborn and premature infant ranges

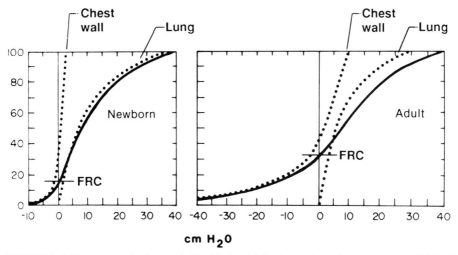

FIGURE 2-1. The pressure/volume relationship (static) for the total respiratory system (solid line), chest wall, and lungs of the infant compared with those of the adult. The end expiratory balance point occurs where the respiratory system curve crosses the zero line, thus indicating a very low FRC.

from 4.2 to 6.5 ml/cm H_2O/kg body weight, depending on gestational age. By adolescence, compliance is much lower; that is, the chest wall has become more rigid, with compliance measured at 2.5 ml/cm H_2O/kg.

The chest wall actually functions through two forces: the diaphragm, which affects the caudal surface of the lung, and the remainder of the lung, which is driven by the expansion of the rib cage. Depending on the relative compliances of the chest wall and lung, the force of one, to a varying extent, counterbalances the force of the other. Forces such as intercostal muscles, which stabilize the chest wall, improve the efficiency of breathing. Those that destabilize it, such as muscular weakness, cost the infant in increased effort in breathing.

In infants without parenchymal disease, the chest wall is so pliable that diaphragmatic effort tends to collapse the chest wall rather than increase lung volume. To compensate for this lack of structural rigidity, the infant "sets" his chest wall muscles to resist the pull of the diaphragm. If this intercostal muscle activity is impaired by fatigue or pain medication, excessive distortion of the chest wall occurs and the work required to maintain minute ventilation will increase. As rib cage distortion increases, there is an increase in diaphragmatic activity by as much as 450%. Most of the resultant work, however, is done by the rib cage, not the lungs.[6]

The infant lung is relatively stiff, having a compliance of 1 to 2 ml/cm H_2O/ kg. This value decreases further with disease, the best-studied example being respiratory distress syndrome (RDS). In cases of RDS, lung compliance has been measured as low as 0.9 ml/cm H_2O/kg. Similar decreases could be expected from increases in lung water (pulmonary edema) or widespread pneumonia.

In the infant, then, there is a net collapsing (emptying) force on the respiratory system as the lung provides more recoil inward than does the chest wall outward. Passive FRC, the point at which the inward and outward forces balance each other, results in a resting lung volume very near residual volume (RV), or at about 15% of total lung capacity (TLC) (see Fig. 2–1). Compare this value with that of the adult, in whom the resting point results in a lung volume of about 30% TLC.

The infant compensates for low passive FRC by the phenomenon of inspiratory muscle braking during exhalation, an activity characterized by starting inspiration before passive exhalation is completed and before lung volume has fallen too close to RV. Measured FRC during active tidal breathing in infants is approximately 35% of TLC, similar to the adult value. A second factor in maintaining FRC is the high respiratory rate in infants. When combined with an airway time constant of 1 second, the accelerated respiratory rate prevents the infant lung from reaching passive FRC by limiting the volume of air expelled during passive exhalation. Disruption of this process by drugs or spontaneous apnea results in a very low lung volume and a decrement in gas exchange.

The closing volume of the lung affects oxygenation as well as low passive FRC. If a child breathes below closing capacity, as can happen during sleep, oxygenation will fall as more airways close and a greater percentage of pulmonary blood flow bypasses well-ventilated alveoli. Infants have a high closing volume, which decreases until 16 years of age. Because infant airways close at high lung volume, a greater degree of ventilation perfusion imbalance occurs than if closing volume were at low lung volume. Closing volume appears to follow a pattern reciprocal to that of elastic recoil (Fig. 2–2).

The dynamics of breathing in the infant are important as well. The infant diaphragm must contract with sufficient force and frequency to compensate for the deficiencies in respiratory system mechanics previously described. These imbalances are more pronounced in disease states, and, consequently, the diaphragm is required to work more when a child is ill. The infant diaphragm differs from that of an adult in that it contains more fast oxidative, fatigue-sensi-

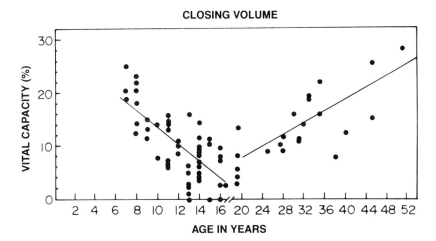

CLOSING VOLUME

Closing volume - The volume of gas remaining in
the vital capacity at the
intersection of phases III + IV
of the closing volume test.
Usually expressed as % of VC
(CV/VC, %)

Closing capacity - The amount of gas remaining
in the total lung capacity is CV + RV.
Usually expressed as a percent of TLC
(CC/TLC, %).

FIGURE 2–2. Phase IV of the single breath oxygen or closing volume test. If closing capacity is greater than FRC, alveolar units will close during tidal breathing, thereby reducing gas exchange. (From Mansell A, Bryan C, Levison H: Airway closure in children. J Appl Physiol 33(6):711–714, 1972.)

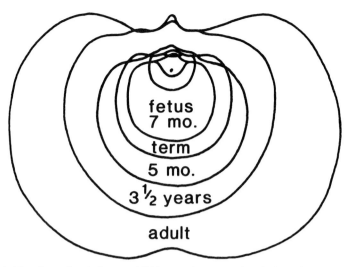

FIGURE 2–3. The chest of an infant or child is round compared with that of an adult. This round shape confers a mechanical advantage to the infant during inspiration. (From Kendig EL, Chernick V: Disorders of the Respiratory Tract, 4th ed. Philadelphia, WB Saunders, 1983.)

tive fibers (Type IIa fibers) and a lower proportion of fatigue-resistant fibers (Type I fibers). This ratio results in a muscle that is more prone to fatigue under prolonged work loads.

The configuration of the diaphragm in the chest does provide, under normal circumstances, some advantage to the infant. The infant diaphragm has a greater curve and maintains a higher position in the thorax than does the adult diaphragm. Its shape and position give the infant the advantage of a more favorable length-tension ratio and permit a higher pressure to be generated for a given contraction (explained by the La Place relationship [$P = 2T/r$]). The shape of the chest wall in infants also augments the contraction of the diaphragm. Owing to the angle of insertion of the diaphragmatic fibers into the lower ribs and the angle of articulation of the ribs, the ribs are lifted cephalad by diaphragmatic contraction. The volume change resulting from this displacement of the ribs is greater in the infant than in the adult because of the larger relative anteroposterior (AP) diameter of the infant's thorax (Fig. 2–3). This configuration, which results in a bucket handle effect, spares work for the infant's diaphragm.

Unfortunately, these advantages are usually negated if the infant develops obstruction in the airways and subsequent air trapping occurs. The diaphragm is then depressed and the ribs elevated by the hyperexpanded lung. These developments negate the benefits of a highly curved diaphragm and rounded chest.

Abdominal contents and the extent to which they restrict the movement of the chest wall and elevate the diaphragm affect a child's breathing effectiveness. Martin and colleagues measured transcutaneous oxygen in 16 preterm infants in supine and prone positions.[5] Strain gauges were used to measure abdominal and chest wall movement. They found that PaO_2 increased in the prone position by 7.4 mmHg, or 15% of the value in the supine position, a significant amount. In five infants with cardiopulmonary disease, the increase was 25%. This improvement in PaO_2 was related to a reduction in asynchronous movement of the chest and abdomen. Placement in the prone position, in fact, may be an important therapeutic intervention in infants with marginal respiratory status and may prevent the need for mechanically assisted ventilation.

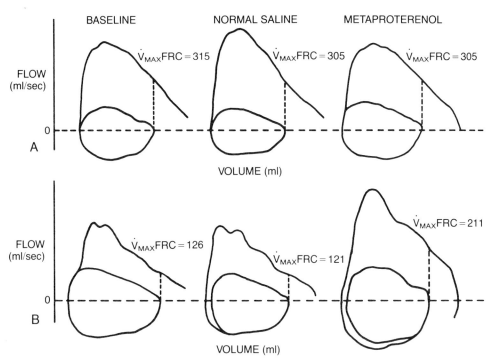

FIGURE 2-4. *A,* The partial flow volume curve shows a large flow reserve at FRC in normal infants. *B,* In infants with a history of wheezing, flow is reduced at FRC, yielding less reserve. These flows can be improved by the bronchodilator metaproterenol, but not by a saline control.

In infants requiring mechanical assistance, prone positioning with the abdomen unsupported improves oxygenation and dynamic compliance. In one group of infants studied when they were recovering from neonatal respiratory disease, mean PaO_2 rose from 70 to 81 mmHg as a result of prone positioning.[11] Whether the difficulties of maintaining and providing nursing care in this position are sufficiently outweighed by the respiratory benefits derived would need to be assessed in each individual case.

The infant's marginally effective respiratory system is further compromised by high airway resistance. Airway resistance in the neonate is apportioned differently within the respiratory system than it is in the adult. In the adult, more than 50% of airway resistance is contributed by the nose. In infants, however, the nose contributes only about one third of the resistance, with the lower airways contributing more to total resistance than they do in the adult. These figures ring true when one considers that the infant, if not an obligate nose-breather, is certainly forced to breathe nasally when feeding; a lower nasal resistance would make this task easier. Similarly, it is known that airway resistance is related to lung volume, resistance increasing rapidly as absolute lung volume decreases. As can be seen in Figure 2–4, this is not a straight line function; resistance climbs at a greater rate at the lowest volumes. As a result, the infant's absolute resistance is higher and also changes more dramatically as lung volume falls.

Airway resistance itself is partitioned in such a way that the small airways contribute more to total resistance in the infant (50%) than in the adult (20%). The change to the adult pattern occurs around 5 years of age and is different in males than in females. The high small airway resistance in infants may contribute to the poor performance of smaller infants stricken with a small airway dis-

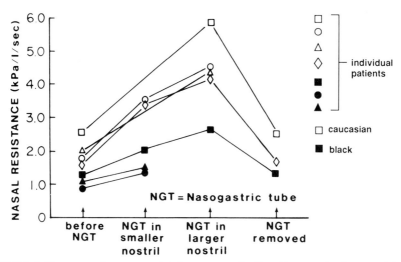

FIGURE 2–5. Placement of a nasogastric tube causes a significant increase in airway resistance in infants. (Reprinted with permission from Stocks J: Effect of nasogastric tubes on nasal resistance during infancy. Arch Dis Child 55:17–21, 1980.)

ease. Bronchiolitis, for instance, can result in a 200 to 300% increase in total respiratory system resistance in infants, while leaving the respiratory mechanics in adults essentially unchanged.

Flaring of the alae nasi may contribute to a reduction in nasal resistance and stabilization of the airway. Carlo and coworkers showed that phasic alae nasi activity occurred with 43% of the breaths during active sleep versus 14% during quiet sleep.[3] Resistance during those breaths accompanied by nasal flaring was, on average, 20% lower in both active and quiet sleep. The authors concluded that alae nasi activity may be important in facilitating ventilation by reducing nasal resistance; it also may help to stabilize the upper airway by preventing the development of large negative pharyngeal pressure during inspiration, a factor that would subsequently have a collapsing effect on the airway.

One must assume that a procedure or medication that impairs alae nasi activity may result in increased effort during breathing and potentiate obstructive apnea. The effect of nasogastric tube placement on nasal resistance in infants has been assessed by Stocks.[9] Nasal resistance increased by 101% in white infants and 50% in black infants when the nasogastric tube was passed through the smaller nostril. There appears to be some compensation, however, as total airways resistance rose less than nasal resistance (Fig. 2–5). Placement of a nasogastric tube, then, can have a profound effect on airway mechanics and should be considered carefully, especially in infants with lung disease. It is for this reason that we prefer to use orogastric tubes in infants during the developmental period, at which time they are obligate nose-breathers. This period usually lasts until 3 to 6 months of age, corrected for abbreviated or lengthy gestation.

Clinical experience with infants suffering from unilateral choanal atresia reveals that these infants become extremely distressed if the patent naris is obstructed by secretions or a nasogastric tube. It has recently been shown that infants can breathe through their mouths if the nose is obstructed; in clinical situations, however, this switch to mouth-breathing does not seem to be efficient, and nasal obstruction can certainly cause severe respiratory distress.

CLINICAL SIGNS OF RESPIRATORY FAILURE

The infant, who has little respiratory reserve, attempts to maximize efficiency by altering his or her pattern of breathing. As distress increases, inspiratory flow increases and inspiratory time (Ti) is reduced. This activity leads to an increase in the work of breathing. The higher respiratory rate causes a shortening of both Ti and expiratory time (TE). The work of breathing is further increased, and the recovery time of the skeletal muscles during exhalation is lessened, the latter hastening the onset of respiratory muscle fatigue. The infant respiratory pattern consequently becomes very rapid and shallow, and respiration becomes disorganized as the chest wall and abdominal wall become asynchronous and then paradoxical. If this pattern is allowed to continue, it is followed by periodic respiratory pauses that do not last long enough to be called apnea events but are clearly noticeable in an infant whose respiratory drive is high. These pauses are presumed to allow for short periods of metabolic recovery for the tiring diaphragm and, as such, indicate severe muscle fatigue.

PHYSICAL SIGNS OF RESPIRATORY DISTRESS

The physical signs of respiratory distress are characterized by increased nasal flaring and retraction of the suprasternal, intercostal, and substernal soft tissues. The observer should remember that recession of the lower intercostal spaces is normal and caused by a slight negative pressure at these points as the diaphragm peels off the chest wall. Owing to the softness of the chest wall in the neonate, retractions, especially those of the substernal variety, may become quite dramatic and result in a great deal of wasted energy as the chest wall, instead of air, is sucked in.

A sign of dyspnea exclusive to infants is the head bob. With the head supported only in the occipital region, it can be seen to bob forward with each breath. This activity is thought to be the effect of the scalene and sternocleidomastoid muscles contracting as accessory muscles of inspiration. In the older child, this contraction helps to stabilize the chest wall and raise the sternum and the first two ribs. When the contraction is unopposed by the neck extensor muscles, the head is pulled down and bobs while the ribs remain unelevated.

Many of the physical signs of respiratory distress result from vigorous contraction of the muscles of respiration, both inspiratory and expiratory. These signs cannot be produced by infants and children with neuromuscular disorders owing to the weak nature of the contractions generated by failing muscles. Such a child may be experiencing respiratory failure but may appear quiet and calm to the observer. Diaphoresis or an anxious appearance may be the only clue to the infant's distress.

In the case of infants with expiratory air flow obstruction, the abdominal musculature can be seen and felt to be contracting with every respiratory cycle, thus adding to the metabolic cost of respiration.

CLEANSING MECHANISMS

The effective cough is an important cleansing mechanism for the pediatric airway. The generation of forces promoting high velocities and large air volume during the cough is dependent on the patency of airways, the strength of the expiratory muscles, and the infant's ability to close the glottis. Operative procedures that interfere with expiratory musculature or chest mechanics and the presence of an endotracheal tube or tracheostomy reduce cough effectiveness.

Ciliary function also contributes to the normal cleansing mechanism of the airway. Although diseases that impair ciliary function are rare (cystic fibrosis, dysmotile cilia syndrome, and Kartagener's syndrome, to name a few), some medications and therapies may decrease it. Barbiturates reduce ciliary activity and may predispose to retention of secretions with resultant pneumonia, especially if they are used for long periods. Oxygen has a dose/time-dependent negative effect on cilial activity; long-term use of high concentrations of oxygen can result in squamous metaplasia of ciliated epithelium, a condition that results in a loss of cilia and, accordingly, their function. The contribution that this loss of function makes to the incidence of nosocomial respiratory infections in infants is not clear, but careful consideration must be made before such medications are prescribed.

CONGENITAL MALFORMATIONS

Infants with underlying lung disease for whom surgical procedures are indicated present a challenge for the pediatric surgeon. These children have congenital malformations of the respiratory system that present as clinical problems in four primary ways: breathlessness, recurrent infection, wheezing, and incidental findings on chest x-ray.

In general, breathlessness, tachypnea, and respiratory distress are the result of altered pulmonary mechanics. The degree of distress is related to the size of the congenital lesion and the extent of its disruption of respiratory function. If they are large in size, cystic adenomatoid malformations and various forms of lung cysts tend to interfere with respiration early in life. Intrapulmonary cysts may rupture, causing pneumothorax, but this complication is unusual. These cysts may, however, enlarge and cause compression of normal lung tissue with increased distress. This action, enlargement without decompression, is the result of a flap-valve effect caused by the collapse of airways not supported by cartilage.

Operation is indicated for all cysts causing respiratory distress. The surgical outcome should be the restoration of respiratory mechanics to near normal following the immediate postoperative period. If large portions of the lung are removed, however, the child may eventually develop a scoliosis, which, in turn, may slightly impair respiratory function.

In congenital lobar emphysema (CLE), the involved lobe is uniformly distended. The affected infant typically presents in the first few months of life with tachypnea, intercostal retractions, and intermittent cyanosis. The child may also wheeze on expiration. Rather than bronchospasm, these symptoms may be a product of airway torsion or dynamic compression.

The degree of distress is proportional to the amount of lung compressed; as such, lobectomy may be indicated for persistent respiratory distress in infants. The early intraoperative period may be especially difficult owing to the fact that forceful, positive pressure ventilation can cause an increase in the size of the emphysematous lobe and, consequently, an intensification of the pressure exerted on surrounding structures. Exclusion by selective bronchial intubation may allow the affected lung to return to normal.

At operation, pressure is relieved once the affected lobe is delivered through

EXTRATHORACIC OBSTRUCTION

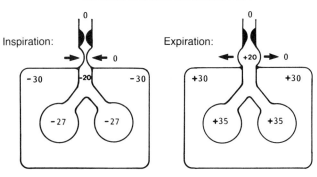

INTRATHORACIC OBSTRUCTION

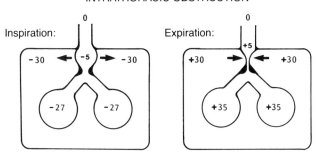

FIGURE 2–6. Airway dynamics during inspiration and expiration. These pressure relationships explain why lesions in different parts of the airway produce symptoms in different phases of respiration.

the thoracotomy incision. The infant should have little postoperative difficulty as the compressed lung reinflates. In approximately 10% of the patients, there will be a recurrence of symptoms due to a second hyperinflated lobe or segment, a condition that, at times, may require further surgical intervention. In fact, lung function testing later in life has shown an obstruction to airflow, indicating that CLE may be a manifestation of widespread pulmonary abnormality.

There are a number of lesions that cause airway obstruction or, more often, partial obstruction. These lesions dramatically affect the mechanics of respiration and the work of breathing. Although they are covered in greater depth elsewhere in this text, the lesions bear mentioning here.

Lesions of the extrathoracic trachea generally result in an expiratory noise as the airways are compressed by the increasing intrathoracic pressure during exhalation (Fig. 2–6). Lesions that cause inspiratory distress may be congenital, such as a subglottic web or hemangioma, or acquired, either from infectious causes such as viral croup or epiglottitis, which is rarely seen in infancy, or from iatrogenic causes such as subglottic stenosis from prolonged intubation of the trachea.

Viral croup affects the upper airway by causing a swelling in the tissues of the subglottic space. Once thought to be due to a tropism of the virus for this area, viral croup has since been shown to affect the entire tracheobronchial tree. Symptoms are primarily related to upper airway obstruction and result in a collapsing force on the trachea as the infant inspires. Severe respiratory distress results, and immediate medical intervention is required.

We have reduced the need for intubation in infants suffering from viral croup by first trying to increase airflow past the stenotic area by having the patient inhale a mixture of 70% helium and 30% oxygen. Because flow past the narrowed segment is turbulent and, as such, dependent upon gas density, reducing the gas density by replacing nitrogen with helium in the breathing mixture increases the gas flow past the obstruction. This action reduces distress and often avoids the need for endotracheal intubation.

The pathophysiology of viral croup extends beyond the upper airway to affect the lower airways as well. Newth and associates have demonstrated that the majority of children with croup are hypoxemic and that the reduction in oxygenation in these infants is the result not of hypoventilation but of ventilation perfusion mismatch.[7]

Congenital lesions such as tracheal webs and hemangiomata produce point lesions, which also obstruct the airway. The collapsing forces within the airway increase as the size of the remaining airway decreases. Patients who suffer from this condition do respond to helium-oxygen mixtures, but the lesion must be removed or bypassed for adequate relief of the airway obstruction. It is important to remember that the greater the inspiratory muscle force generated by the infant, the greater the collapsing force on the airway and chest wall. We recommend, therefore, that infants with stenoses of the trachea be disturbed as little as possible. If left undisturbed, they will naturally adopt the most efficient breathing pattern in terms of rate, force, and timing of inspiration and expiration. Once an adequate airway has been established, a thorough evaluation can be undertaken.

Tracheomalacia and bronchomalacia are lesions of the intrathoracic airway and, as such, cause problems primarily during the expiratory phase of respiration. On physical examination, expiration is prolonged and results in varying degrees of respiratory distress. In the case of a malacic (soft) segment located near the carina, unilateral or even bilateral overinflation of the lungs may occur and lead to generalized respiratory distress. Conservative therapy, such as continuous positive airway pressure (CPAP), should be pursued in these infants before surgical intervention is sought. CPAP alters the mechanics of respiration by preventing complete collapse of the malacic segment, thereby facilitating the egress of air from beyond the lesion. Infants who otherwise would have required prolonged mechanical ventilation or early operative intervention have been sent home successfully on simple CPAP valves.

It is expected that, with growth of the airway, the malacic segment will strengthen and cause less obstruction at normal intrathoracic pressures. In some cases, however, temporary tracheostomy may be necessary.

A number of skeletal anomalies result in changes in chest wall mechanics. Asphyxiating thoracic dystrophy is characterized by extreme narrowing of the rib cage and constriction of the thorax with short ribs. This condition results in a purely restrictive disease in which the chest wall configuration limits lung expansion. Spinal deformities such as scoliosis can cause similar mechanical changes.

Limitations on thoracic cage mobility caused by spinal deformities result in a reduction of TLC and RV. The most economical respiratory pattern is one of rapid, low-volume breaths; when these skeletal deformities are present, adequate air velocities for an effective cough cannot be developed. The result is retention of secretions and infection, both of which cause further restrictive disease. A child with skeletal restriction may require ventilatory support until attempts to repair or stabilize the lesion can be made. The goal is to aid in

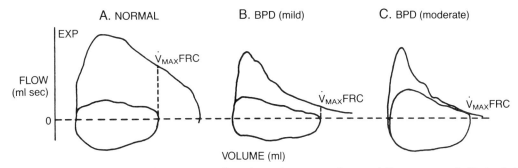

FIGURE 2-7. Infants with BPD can have severe airflow obstruction yet remain essentially asymptomatic *(B)*. A relatively minor disruption to respiratory mechanics can lead to significant deterioration. In both mild (asymptomatic) and moderate (symptomatic) BPD, little flow reserve exists at FRC.

expansion of the chest beyond the point at which the infant's musculature is capable of moving the chest wall. In other words, some method of intermittent positive pressure ventilation (IPPV) is used. In this manner, secretions that would otherwise accumulate can be cleared.

A new understanding of respiratory mechanics in infants is derived from the testing of infant lung function. This testing, now more widely available in pediatric pulmonary function laboratories, is useful in diagnosing infant respiratory disease. There is still, however, a great deal to be learned about the methodology of the tests and their limitations.

One method of testing involves the use of a squeeze technique to produce a maximum flow envelope over the range of tidal breathing. To accomplish this, the infant is tested when sleeping, either naturally or after a small dose of chloral hydrate. The child is wrapped in an inflatable cuff that covers the chest and abdomen, and airflow is measured by placing a low dead space mask over the face and connecting an appropriate pneumotachograph. The signal is recorded on an oscilloscope for photography and measurement; more sophisticated systems allow for computerized acquisition of the signal. The child breathes tidally. At the end of tidal inspiration, the encircling bag is inflated, causing a forceful exhalation and generating a flow-volume curve over the range of tidal breathing (Fig. 2–7). To compare curves, maximum flows at FRC (V̇max FRC) are measured.

Lesions that result in airflow obstruction will reduce flows at FRC and cause the flow-volume curve to be concave. A fixed tracheal lesion may reduce flow to such an extent that the top of the curve is flattened. The augmentation of flow by this technique lasts only 0.5 to 1.0 second, and the baby usually sleeps through the entire procedure.

As can be seen in Figure 2–7, infants with bronchopulmonary dysplasia (BPD) can have significant airflow obstruction with little or no reserve flow beyond that necessary to maintain tidal breathing. These infants, even if free of clinical symptoms, may encounter problems as a result of surgical intervention for other conditions. Their lack of respiratory reserve prevents them from compensating well for fever, pain, or excessive secretions. In infants with BPD, infant lung function testing can be useful in predicting the likelihood of postoperative problems such as the need for prolonged ventilatory support.

Infant lung function testing can also be directed at the effects of medication, such as bronchodilators, on infants with BPD. It has been concluded in earlier studies that infants with airflow obstruction do not respond to inhaled bronchodilators. These results, however, may have been due to a number of factors: the tested population was perhaps too severely affected or the testing methods used were not sensitive enough to discern changes in airway function. Using the squeeze or forced exhalation technique described previously, Tepper and colleagues[10] have shown that flows at FRC ($\dot{V}$max FRC) can be improved by inhaled bronchodilators in infants suffering from viral lower respiratory infection and in those with BPD. This information on the mechanics of airway reactivity is extremely valuable; it allows for the testing of individual infants for responsiveness to bronchodilator drugs and provides scientific validity for the clinical use of aerosolized bronchodilators in the management of infants with respiratory problems.

If infant lung function studies are unavailable or impractical, the effectiveness of bronchodilators is judged by careful clinical evaluation. Generally, however, we at Riley Children's Hospital find that infant lung function studies are quite helpful in the management of infants with respiratory disease. We advocate their use, particularly in infants with chronic disease such as BPD, who may require surgery during infancy.

BPD is a chronic lung disease frequently encountered in the specialized practice of the pediatric surgeon. Although it is not clearly defined, BPD, first described by Northway and coworkers in 1967,[8] is most frequently used to describe infants who were born prematurely and who have evidence of chronic lung disease at 1 month of age.

The incidence of BPD among premature survivors appears to be 20 to 25%. The disease has a wide clinical spectrum; some infants are overtly symptomatic, requiring ventilatory assistance, supplementary oxygen, and chronic medication, whereas others only become symptomatic with a respiratory insult or lower respiratory viral infection. The most severe problems may arise in the least symptomatic infants. These children have clearly abnormal lung function when tested but are without symptoms; as such, they may not receive sufficient pre- and postsurgical attention.

Respiratory dysfunction may be precipitated by the stresses relative to a surgical procedure such as fluid shifts, pain, and disruption of the muscles of inspiratory and expiratory respiration. Using the clinically available techniques described, the pediatric pulmonologist can now test the lung function of these infants and determine the degree of impairment. Studies in BPD infants have demonstrated both an increase in pulmonary and airways resistance and a reduced compliance. Partial expiratory flow-volume curves show low flows at FRC (see Fig. 2–7) and limited flows even at tidal breathing. Other BPD infants, although not limited at tidal flow rates, have no reserve and subsequently are unable to increase respiratory airflow in response to stress. It is important to reiterate that these infants may not be symptomatic until they endure a stressful event requiring an increase in flow at FRC.

Studies of infants recovering from lower respiratory infection and those with asthma (wheezy bronchitis or asthmatic bronchitis) or cystic fibrosis clearly demonstrate that even newborns can respond to inhaled bronchodilators.[4] In the past, the assumption had been made that infants did not have the capability to respond to beta agonist bronchodilators. An increase has now been shown in airflow at FRC ($\dot{V}$max FRC) in infants after inhalation of metaproterenol (see Fig. 2–4). In children with underlying airway disease, the preoperative use of beta agonists may increase flows to improve the infant's cough effectiveness and prevent postoperative complications such as atelectasis.

The infant respiratory system functions adequately in the healthy baby but has little reserve to cope with disruption from disease. Small airways and a highly compliant chest wall contribute to the problem. Even a minor intervention can cause the work of breathing to increase to such an extent that the mechanics of the system cannot compensate. Consequently, consideration of these factors in the planning of an infant's surgery and postoperative care can result in an improved outcome for the patient with less chance of ventilatory failure.

REFERENCES

1. Agostoni E: Volume-pressure relationships of the thorax and lung in the newborn. J Appl Physiol 14:909–913, 1959
2. Avery M, Cook C: Volume-pressure relationship of lungs and thorax in fetal, newborn, and adult goats. J Appl Physiol 16:1034–1038, 1961
3. Carlo WA, et al: Alae nasi—activation (nasal flaring) decreases nasal resistance in preterm infants. Pediatrics 72:338–343, 1983
4. Hiatt P, et al: Bronchodilator response in infants with cystic fibrosis. Am Rev Respir Dis 127:213, 1983
5. Martin RJ, et al: Effect of supine and prone positions on arterial oxygen tension in the preterm infant. Pediatrics 63:528–531, 1979
6. Muller NG, et al: Diaphragmatic muscle fatigue in the newborn. J Appl Physiol 46:688–695, 1979
7. Newth CJL, Levinson H, Bryam AC: The respiratory status of children with croup. J Pediatr 81:206–208, 1972
8. Northway W, Rosen R, Porter D: Pulmonary disease following respiratory therapy of hyaline membrane disease. N Engl J Med 276:357, 1967
9. Stocks J: Effect of nasogastric tubes on nasal resistance during infancy. Arch Dis Child 55:17–21, 1980
10. Tepper R, et al: Forced expiratory flow in infants: A simple non-invasive test of airways obstruction in infants with bronchopulmonary dysplasia. Am Rev Respir Dis 127:213, 1983
11. Wagaman MJ, et al: Improved oxygenation and lung compliance with prone positioning of neonates. J Pediatr 94:787–791, 1979

chapter 3

Radiologic Aspects of Airway Obstruction

Roderick I. Macpherson, M.D.

The airway is the conduit through which air is exchanged between the atmosphere and the alveoli. It has been divided into two main parts: the upper airway (proximal or large airways) and the lower airway (distal or small airways). In this chapter, we are concerned only with the upper airway and consider it to extend from the nose to the mainstem bronchi. Obstructions along this pathway are common and present serious problems in infants and children. There are many potential causes for pediatric airway obstruction, and a variety of diagnostic procedures may be used in their investigation. The radiologist must be fully aware of the pathologic possibilities and undertake an efficient, if not rapid, line of investigation. We review here the radiologic features of the major causes of upper airway obstruction in children and the radiologic techniques that may be used in their investigation.

RADIOLOGIC INVESTIGATIVE PROCEDURES

Standard frontal and lateral radiographs of the chest should be part of the radiologic investigation of all children suspected of having airway obstruction. In many cases, these radiographs are able to demonstrate the cause of the obstruction, offer clues for further investigation, and rule out complications involving the lungs, mediastinum, and pleura. If a check-valve obstruction, such as an intrabronchial foreign body, is suspected, an expiration frontal view of the chest or chest fluoroscopy may be included as well.[42] As an alternative, lateral decubitus views of the chest may be used to achieve the same purpose.

The child who presents with acute respiratory distress characterized by stridor should receive an examination of the soft tissues of the neck to exclude

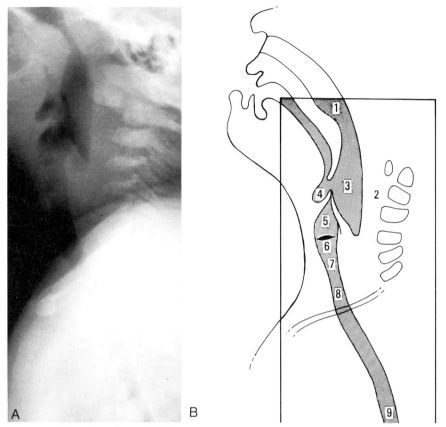

FIGURE 3–1. Normal magnification lateral view of airway. Radiograph (*A*) and corresponding line drawing (*B*) show the anatomic areas that compose the airway: *1,* nasopharynx; *2,* retropharynx; *3,* oropharynx; *4,* valleculae; *5,* supraglottic region; *6,* glottis; *7,* subglottic trachea; *8,* cervical trachea; *9,* intrathoracic trachea. (*A* reprinted with permission from Macpherson RI, Leithiser RE: Upper airway obstruction in children: An update. Radiographics 5:339–376, 1985.)

acute epiglottitis. Of note is the fact that, in cases of acute respiratory emergency, some centers use frontal views of the neck in addition to the lateral projection. My colleagues and I believe that this policy unduly prolongs the desperate child's time in the radiology department, while the films obtained provide little additional information.

The single lateral view of the soft tissues of the neck should be done with the child in the upright position to avoid the life-threatening distress that may develop when a patient with acute epiglottitis is recumbent. The child's chin should be held up and the shoulders down, and the film should be exposed with the child in deep inspiration. This position permits clear visualization of the oropharynx and supraglottic, glottic, and subglottic structures and avoids the spurious widening of the retropharyngeal soft tissues that may occur in expiration or when the head is flexed.

Magnification lateral (Fig. 3–1) and frontal (Fig. 3–2) overhead views of the upper airway, the technical details of which are summarized in Table 3–1, can be done in elective situations.[19] The high kilovoltage technique enhances soft tissue detail, whereas the special filters provide a more uniform density from the nasal passages to the mainstem bronchi. The 2 to 1 magnification makes it easier to view the subtle abnormalities sometimes encountered. Frontal and lateral overhead magnification is a technique that requires planning and practice;

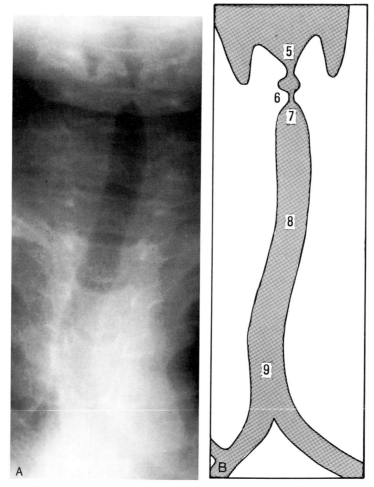

FIGURE 3–2. Normal magnification frontal view of airway. Radiograph (*A*) and corresponding line drawing (*B*) show the component parts of the airway perceptible on this view: *5*, supraglottic region; *6*, glottis; *7*, subglottic trachea; *8*, cervical trachea; *9*, intrathoracic trachea. (*A* reprinted with permission from Macpherson RI, Leithiser RE: Upper airway obstruction in children: An update. Radiographics 5:339–376, 1985.)

TABLE 3–1. Magnification Radiography of the Airway: Technical Considerations

Projections	Anteroposterior and lateral
Position	Supine with head extended
Focal-film distance	60 inches
Object-film distance	30 inches
Magnification	2 to 1
Filtration	Thoraeus filter on AP
Focal spot	0.3 mm
KVP	High (125–135)
maS	Low (1.6–2.5)
Film	Ultra detail, high contrast
Screens	High speed, rare earth

Reprinted with permission from Macpherson RI, Leithiser RE: Upper airway obstruction in children: An update. Radiographics 5:339–376, 1985.

it is not recommended for use in centers that have a small volume of children with airway obstruction or in acute emergency situations.

Videofluoroscopy[22] is an invaluable adjunct to the overhead films. It can be used to study the dynamic changes that take place in the airway during the respiratory cycle: variations in the width of the retropharyngeal soft tissues, movements of the aryepiglottic folds (see Fig. 3–9), and fluctuations in the caliber and position of the trachea (see Fig. 3–30). Videofluoroscopy is very helpful in confirming the presence of airway obstruction suspected on the basis of the overhead magnification films (see Fig. 3–12).

Another part of the initial evaluation of a patient with upper airway obstruction of unknown etiology is the esophagogram, which helps to demonstrate or exclude the presence of vascular rings (see Fig. 3–19), slings (see Fig. 3–20), and mediastinal (see Fig. 3–31) as well as cervical masses. Note that for an esophagogram, the study should include the true lateral position and that fluoroscopy, preferably videofluoroscopy, should be used.

Standard linear or polytomography may occasionally be called upon to provide a clear delineation of problems suspected on the initial films. Tomography is particularly useful in demonstrating the nature and longitudinal extent of tracheal stenoses (see Fig. 3–26B).

Xerography[18] is another method of imaging the upper airway in children. With its edge-enhancement properties, this special technique provides an excellent means by which to study soft tissues and can be used when a demonstration of subtle soft tissue changes is diagnostically important. We have found it useful in evaluating the trachea and mainstem bronchi when, for example, a congenital tracheal stenosis is suspected (see Figs. 3–21 and 3–24).

Tracheography is considered a last resort; it is used only when all other methods of assessing the trachea have proven unsatisfactory. In our experience, when this examination is necessary in very ill, intubated infants it must be performed swiftly. A small amount of thin, bronchographic contrast medium is introduced via the endotracheal tube followed by rapid filming or videofluoroscopy. In addition to an excellent anatomic demonstration of the trachea and mainstem bronchi (see Figs. 3–20B and 3–21B), tracheography also provides an assessment of tracheal dynamics.

Computed tomography (CT) is currently the method of choice in the evaluation of upper airway obstruction when a mass is involved (see Figs. 3–4, 3–5, 3–16, and 3–22).[20,26] CT provides useful information regarding the site, size, nature, and extent of the lesion before treatment.

Magnetic resonance imaging (MRI) is currently being evaluated as a way to image airway obstruction in children.[14,32] Because it is capable of demonstrating the large airways and blood vessels simultaneously and in several planes without using ionizing radiation or contrast media, MRI would seem to be an ideal method. It has, however, received mixed reviews. MRI is capable of demonstrating the vascular-related airway obstruction,[14] but the long imaging time presently required makes it inferior to CT as a method of evaluating mediastinal masses.[32] As the technology improves, however, MRI may become the method of choice in children with certain types of airway obstruction.

Angiography may play an important role in the preoperative evaluation of children suspected of having vascular rings (see Fig. 3–19), pulmonary slings (see Fig. 3–20), or the anomalous innominate artery syndrome (see Fig. 3–17).[35]

Choanography is a simple procedure performed in newborn infants suspected of having choanal atresia or stenosis[39] but can also be used to delineate

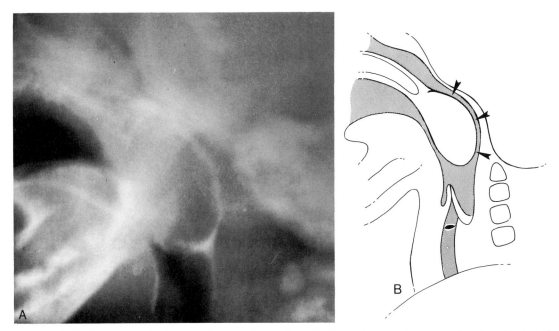

FIGURE 3-3. Benign teratoma in the nasopharynx of a newborn. Radiograph (*A*) and corresponding line drawing (*B*) show a soft tissue mass (arrowheads) in the soft palate outlined during choanography. (*A* reprinted with permission from Macpherson RI, Leithiser RE: Upper airway obstruction in children: An update. Radiographics 5:339–376, 1985.)

other causes of nasal or nasopharyngeal obstruction in neonates (Fig. 3–3). We prefer to perform choanography as a fluoroscopic procedure. As such, we set the fluoroscopic table in the horizontal position and place the infant supine on the elevated foot board. A small amount of contrast medium is then instilled into each of the child's nostrils, and its progress through the nares and into the nasopharynx is observed and recorded. Any contrast medium, including barium, can be used, although we tend to avoid the water-soluble varieties.

Various other radiologic procedures may be called upon if specific causes of airway obstruction are suspected. Isotope studies, for example, can be used to rule out ectopic thyroid as a cause of nasopharyngeal, retropharyngeal, vallecular (see Fig. 3–6), or mediastinal masses. Another distinctive radiologic procedure is the so-called sleep apnea study,[12] a special videofluoroscopic evaluation performed on children suspected of having obstructive sleep apnea. The only difference between the sleep apnea study and the regular fluoroscopic assessment of the airway is that the former is done while the child is sleeping.

RADIOLOGIC FEATURES

The upper airway may be divided into several anatomically distinct sections, each of which is discussed hereafter.

Nares

The nares, or nasal passages, act as the front door to the upper airway and are a seemingly forgotten site of airway obstruction in children. Newborn infants are obligate nose-breathers (see Chapter 2). Consequently, congenital nasopharyngeal obstruction can produce life-threatening apnea, be it complete (atresia) or incomplete (stenosis), unilateral or bilateral.[39] The occluding septum may vary from a thin diaphragm to a thick, bony wall. Choanal atresia or stenosis should be suspected, and later confirmed by choanography, when a catheter cannot be passed through one or both nares. CT has been used to evaluate the nature and thickness of the congenital occlusion.

Nasopharynx

The nasopharynx is that portion of the pharynx situated above the level of the soft palate. Neonatal asphyxia may be the result of airway obstruction due to tumors in this area.[15] Nasopharyngeal teratomas, the most common of these tumors, usually arise from the posterior wall of the nasopharynx and can be recognized on lateral neck radiographs as nasopharyngeal soft tissue masses containing amorphous calicifications and/or bone. These tumors also occasionally arise from the soft palate (see Fig. 3–3) and may be outlined during choanography.

Juvenile angiofibromas are the most common benign tumor of the nasopharynx in older children.[36] They are typically found in teenage males and cause epistaxis and airway obstruction. On lateral views of the neck, these tumors are seen as soft tissue masses that, while impacted in the nasopharynx, displace the posterior walls of the maxillary antra anteriorly. In the past, angiography was used to demonstrate the limits of these highly vascular masses; the current investigation of choice, however, is CT. Using a bolus injection of contrast medium along with rapid sequence scanning, a homogenous enhancement of the tumor can be obtained (Fig. 3–4). Malignant tumors originating in the naso-

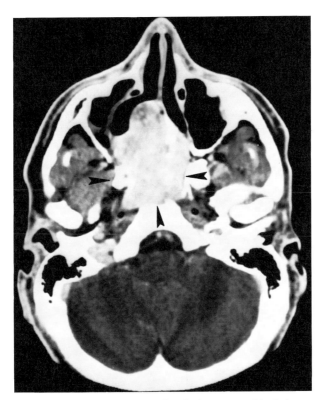

FIGURE 3–4. Juvenile angiofibroma in a teen-aged male demonstrated by bolus contrast CT. Note the intensely enhancing nasopharyngeal mass (arrowheads) displacing the posterior wall of the right maxillary antrum.

pharyngeal region include rhabdomyosarcomas, neuroblastomas, and nasopharyngeal carcinoma.

Enlarged adenoids, which result in either partial or complete occlusion of the nasopharynx, can cause serious hypoventilation in children. This condition leads, in turn, to chronic hypoxemia and hypercapnia with eventual cor pulmonale and neurologic damage,[12] a sequence of events often associated with obstructive sleep apnea. Radiologists can subjectively evaluate adenoidal size on lateral neck films with recognition of a wide normal variation, whereas an objective appraisal can be obtained by using an adenoidal-nasopharyngeal ratio.[16] All measurements aside, however, the adenoids are definitely enlarged if they touch the hard palate.

Retropharyngeal Space

The retropharyngeal space defines the area between the pharynx and the cervical spine. Easily assessed on lateral radiographs of the neck, the retropharyngeal space can measure up to three quarters of the anteroposterior (AP) diameter of adjacent cervical bodies in infants.[20] In older children, however, 3 mm is considered the upper limits of normal width.[38] It should be remembered that the retropharyngeal soft tissues may appear thickened on lateral airway films exposed during expiration or with the neck flexed. This apparent widening should not be confused with a retropharyngeal mass. Fluoroscopy is helpful in making this differentiation.

Masses in the retropharyngeal space can encroach on the oropharyngeal airway and, as a result, cause respiratory distress.[24] The mass most commonly seen in this area is the retropharyngeal abscess (Fig. 3–5), which usually ensues from respiratory tract infections and, less often, from perforating injuries of the pharynx or esophagus. Fever, neck stiffness, and dysphagia are the classic symptoms; occasionally, however, these abscesses will present with signs of airway obstruction. The radiologic features are characteristic: fixed widening and bulging of the retropharyngeal soft tissues, anterior displacement of the airway, and, often, reversal of the normal cervical lordotic curvature. CT (Fig. 3–5C) can be used to confirm the diagnosis of retropharyngeal abscess and demonstrate the size and location of the pus collection before surgical drainage.

Other types of retropharyngeal masses include cystic hygroma, branchial cleft cyst, neuroblastoma, neurofibromatosis, hemangioma, retropharyngeal goiter, and lymph node enlargement of any origin.[24] Of these, cystic hygroma (cavernous lymphangioma) is the most common.[30] These compressible, cystlike, congenital masses usually originate in the posterior cervical triangle; they can, however, extend toward the midline and into the retropharyngeal space and down into the mediastinum as well. CT (see Figs. 3–4 and 3–5) is useful in the preoperative evaluation of all cystic and solid cervical masses.[26]

Oropharynx

The oropharynx is that portion of the pharynx between the soft palate and the epiglottis. It is a link in the airway chain that contains some unexpected mechanisms for airway obstruction. Enlarged tonsils can compromise the oropharynx and cause obstructive sleep apnea. In addition, there are certain craniofacial syndromes in which the tongue, owing to either its position or its size, may

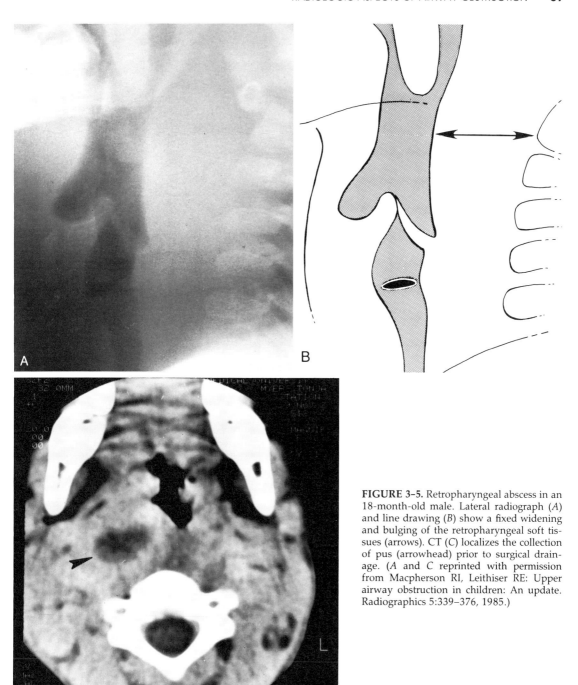

FIGURE 3-5. Retropharyngeal abscess in an 18-month-old male. Lateral radiograph (*A*) and line drawing (*B*) show a fixed widening and bulging of the retropharyngeal soft tissues (arrows). CT (*C*) localizes the collection of pus (arrowhead) prior to surgical drainage. (*A* and *C* reprinted with permission from Macpherson RI, Leithiser RE: Upper airway obstruction in children: An update. Radiographics 5:339–376, 1985.)

obstruct the airway.[38] The best known of these disorders is the Pierre Robin syndrome, in which cleft palate and micrognathia are associated with retroposition of the tongue (glossoptosis). The tongue of the child with Pierre Robin syndrome encroaches on the airway, particularly when the infant is recumbent, causing either acute apneic spells or more chronic symptoms such as obstructive sleep apnea. This phenomenon occurs in other syndromes also associated with

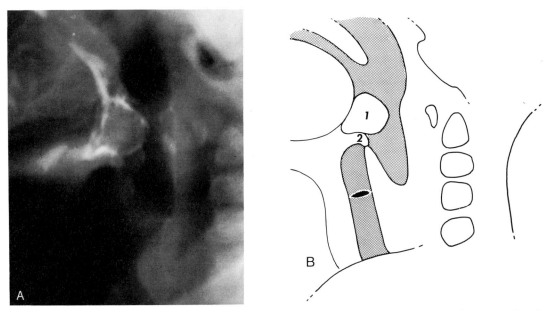

FIGURE 3-6. Ectopic thyroid in the valleculae. A lateral spot film during an esophagogram (*A*) and corresponding line drawing (*B*) show a vallecular mass (*1*), outlined by barium, displacing the epiglottis (*2*) posteriorly, causing airway obstruction. A thyroid scan showed ectopic thyroid. (*A* reprinted with permission from Macpherson RI, Leithiser RE: Upper airway obstruction in children: An update. Radiographics 5:339–376, 1985.)

micrognathia, such as Goldenhar's syndrome and Treacher Collins syndrome. Macroglossia, or a large tongue, is seen in children with cretinism and the Beck-with-Wiedemann syndrome as well as in those with lingular tumors and cysts. Finally, foreign bodies may impact in the infant's oropharynx and cause airway obstruction.

Valleculae

The valleculae are depressions, one on either side of the midline frenulum, located in the valley between the base of the tongue and the epiglottis. Relatively small masses in this area can displace the epiglottis posteroinferiorly into the airway and subsequently cause serious obstruction (Fig. 3–6). A variety of lesions—teratomas, thyroglossal cysts, laryngeal cysts, abscesses, and hematomas—can occur in this area. It is in the valleculae that ectopic thyroid can be found impinging on the airway (see Fig. 3–6),[10] the definitive diagnosis of which can be established by a thyroid isotope scan.

Supraglottic Region

The supraglottic region is located between the epiglottis and the true cords. Most of the lesions in this area are found in the epiglottis and aryepiglottic folds. Acute bacterial epiglottitis, usually due to *Haemophilus influenzae*, produces acute airway obstruction with inflammation and swelling of the epiglottis and aryepiglottic folds.[10] Affected children are usually between 3 and 6 years of age and present with severe respiratory distress characterized by stridor, symptoms similar to those associated with croup and foreign body aspiration. Because the

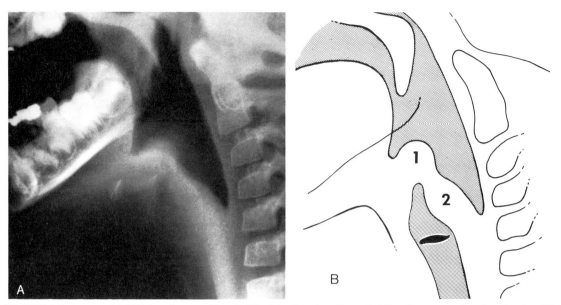

FIGURE 3-7. Acute epiglottitis in a 3-year-old male. The lateral neck radiograph (*A*) and corresponding line drawing (*B*) show the characteristic swelling of the epiglottis (*1*) and aryepiglottic folds (*2*), along with the often associated pharyngeal distension and cervical kyphosis. (*A* reprinted with permission from Macpherson RI, Leithiser RE: Upper airway obstruction in children: An update. Radiographics 5:339–376, 1985.)

differential diagnosis must be made rapidly, a single lateral view of the neck is suggested. With this approach, the characteristic marked swelling of both the epiglottis and the aryepiglottic folds can be clearly visualized (Fig. 3–7). Note that distension of the pharynx and cervical kyphosis are common secondary signs of acute bacterial epiglottitis (see Chapter 4 for clinical management).

Other causes of obstructive inflammatory swelling of the epiglottis and aryepiglottic folds are angioneurotic edema, caustic ingestion, and radiation therapy to the neck. In addition, to complicate matters, there are certain noninflammatory causes of enlargement of the aryepiglottic folds and/or epiglottis that can be confused with acute epiglottitis.[25] Aryepiglottic fold cysts are a type of congenital laryngeal cyst; they occur anywhere along the aryepiglottic folds and can measure up to 2.5 cm in diameter.[31] These cysts usually cause stridor, either at birth or shortly thereafter, and appear as localized smooth swellings of an aryepiglottic fold (Fig. 3–8). Tumors of the aryepiglottic folds are quite uncommon and are usually benign.

Laryngomalacia is the most common cause of neonatal stridor.[34] "Floppy aryepiglottic folds" sag into the airway during inspiration and give rise to a fluttering stridor first noted at birth especially when the infant is supine. This infolding of the aryepiglottic folds is presumably due to immaturity of the supportive cartilaginous structures. The diagnosis can be made by videofluoroscopy (Fig. 3–9), but treatment is rarely required because infants commonly outgrow the problem within the first 18 months of life.

Glottis

The glottis is defined as the true vocal cords and the space that lies between them. A few obstructing lesions, the congenital causes of which are laryngeal

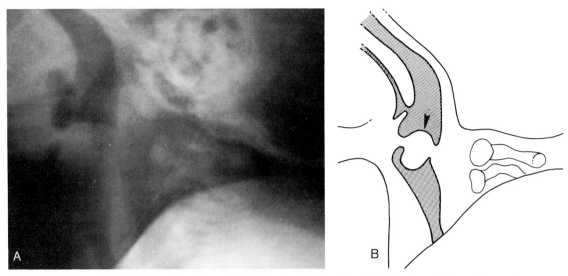

FIGURE 3-8. Aryepiglottic fold cyst in a 5-month-old female with chronic stridor. The lateral view of the neck (*A*) and line drawing (*B*) show a rounded, soft tissue mass in the area of the aryepiglottic folds (arrowhead). This was more clearly delineated by fluoroscopy and esophagography prior to surgery. (*A* reprinted with permission from Macpherson RI, Leithiser RE: Upper airway obstruction in children: An update. Radiographics 5:339–376, 1985.)

atresia, laryngeal stenosis, and laryngeal webs occur at this level. Congenital laryngeal webs, the most common cause of obstructing lesions within the glottis,[34] are bands of varying thickness. The webs are usually located anteriorly at the level of the cores and obliterate the anterior commissure; they occasionally occur just below the true cords but are rarely seen above them. Associated with a weak or absent cry and varying degrees of stridor and respiratory distress, the webs can be a cause of severe airway obstruction and are often found in conjunction with other anomalies such as congenital subglottic stenosis. Congenital laryngeal webs can be seen on lateral airway films; CT, however, may provide more precise information concerning their exact location, size, and associated anomalies.

Laryngeal papillomatosis is the most common type of laryngeal tumor in children.[7] Primarily affecting the glottis, these lesions are numerous and cause progressive hoarseness and stridor. On airway films, laryngeal papillomas appear as irregular filling defects in the glottic region (Fig. 3–10). They can seed peripherally in the respiratory tract and result in pulmonary nodules or nonspecific parenchymal changes, either of which can eventually lead to chronic pulmonary disease and death. Although the etiology of laryngeal papillomatosis is not fully understood, a viral cause is highly probable. Many methods of treatment exist. None, however, has proven completely successful, and recurrences are very common.

Trachea

The trachea, which extends from the glottis to the carina, is the longest portion of the upper airway. For the purposes of this discussion, it is subdivided into three parts: the subglottic trachea, the cervical trachea, and the intrathoracic trachea.

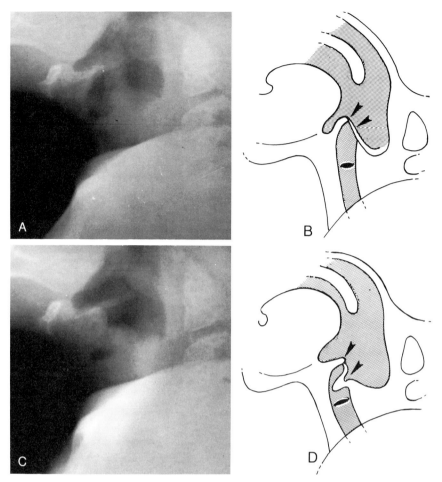

FIGURE 3–9. Laryngomalacia in an infant with stridor. The radiograph (*A*) and line drawing (*B*) of the lateral airway show the normal appearance of the epiglottis and aryepiglottic folds (arrowheads) on expiration. The radiograph (*C*) and corresponding line drawing (*D*) show an anterior and inferior bowing of these structures (arrowheads) during inspiration. At fluoroscopy a fluttering of the folds coincident with the stridor is frequently perceptible. (*B* and *D* reprinted with permission from Macpherson RI, Leithiser RE: Upper airway obstruction in children: An update. Radiographics 5:339–376, 1985.)

SUBGLOTTIC TRACHEA

The subglottic trachea is the short tracheal segment between the undersurface of the true vocal cords and the inferior margin of the cricoid cartilage. It is the narrowest portion of the child's airway; as such, relatively minor degrees of mucosal or submucosal thickening in this area may cause serious airway obstruction.

Croup, or acute laryngotracheobronchitis,[8] is a viral inflammation involving the larynx and trachea diffusely. The classic clinical presentation of fever, "brassy" cough, and acute stridor in children 6 months to 3 years of age is usually sufficient to make the diagnosis. Airway studies, however, are occasionally requested to exclude acute epiglottitis and other causes of acute stridor. If time is of the essence—in an emergency situation, for instance—a single lateral view of the upper airway can be used to exclude epiglottitis and demonstrate the

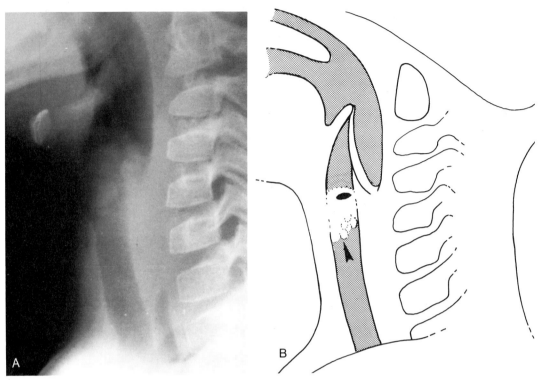

FIGURE 3-10. Laryngeal papillomatosis in a 4-year-old female with chronic stridor and hoarseness. The lateral radiograph of the neck (*A*) and corresponding line drawing (*B*) show irregular polypoid defects on the glottis (arrowhead) consistent with papillomatosis. (*A* reprinted with permission from Macpherson RI, Leithiser RE: Upper airway obstruction in children: An update. Radiographics 5:339–376, 1985.)

subglottic edema consistent with croup. Radiologic signs of croup, however, can be seen on both frontal (Fig. 3–11) and lateral (Fig. 3–12) airway films (see Chapter 4 for clinical discussion).

Frontal films of the child with croup reveal a loss of the normal "shouldering" of the air column below the true cords with replacement by a tapered appearance or "steeple sign" (see Fig. 3–11). This change can often be seen on the plain chest radiograph (we generally do not include the frontal view in our emergency protocol for children with acute stridor). On the lateral view of the airway (see Fig. 3–12), the subglottic trachea is narrow and indistinct. Distension of the hypopharynx on inspiration and the cervical trachea on expiration is fluoroscopic evidence of airway obstruction at this level.

Subglottic stenosis, either congenital or acquired, may mimic croup both clinically and radiologically. The normally narrow subglottic trachea, affected by congenital subglottic stenosis, is further reduced in width by a circumferential cartilaginous and soft tissue deformity. In severe cases, infants experience respiratory distress with stridor at birth; in milder cases, children suffer recurrent, crouplike episodes during which minor degrees of mucosal edema cause critical airway narrowing.

Acquired subglottic stenosis is usually the result of prolonged endotracheal intubation. Approximately 5% of neonates intubated for respiratory distress syndrome are reported to develop chronic subglottic stenosis. A product of mechanical, chemical, and bacterial irritation to the mucosa in this narrowest

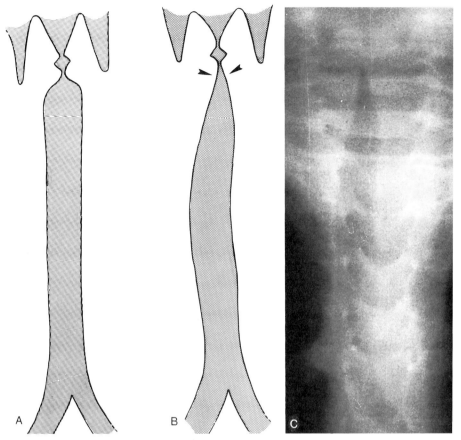

FIGURE 3-11. Croup in a 3-year-old child with acute stridor. Line drawings of the normal frontal appearance of the trachea (*A*) and that associated with croup (*B*) are accompanied by a radiograph with croup (*C*). Note the tapering of the subglottic trachea (arrowheads) compared with the normal. This is referred to as the "steeple sign" of croup. (*C* reprinted with permission from Macpherson RI, Leithiser RE: Upper airway obstruction in children: An update. Radiographics 5: 339–376, 1985.)

segment of the airway, the stenosis may appear on airway studies made immediately following extubation or develop weeks later (Fig. 3–13).

Congenital subglottic hemangioma is a distinct clinical entity[4] and can cause crouplike symptoms that are intermittent at first but become persistent with time. Airway studies of affected children reveal an irregular, small, soft tissue mass below the true vocal cords.

Subglottic mucoceles or mucus retention cysts are a rare complication of prolonged endotracheal intubation.[9] On airway studies (Fig. 3–14), subglottic mucoceles can either have an irregular appearance similar to that of subglottic hemangiomas or may appear as smoothly rounded subglottic filling defects.

CERVICAL AND INTRATHORACIC TRACHEA

The cervical trachea, which extends from the cricoid cartilage to the thoracic inlet, and the intrathoracic trachea, which stretches from the thoracic inlet to the carina, are generally subject to the same diseases and will be considered together as the "trachea." The tracheal causes of upper airway obstruction in

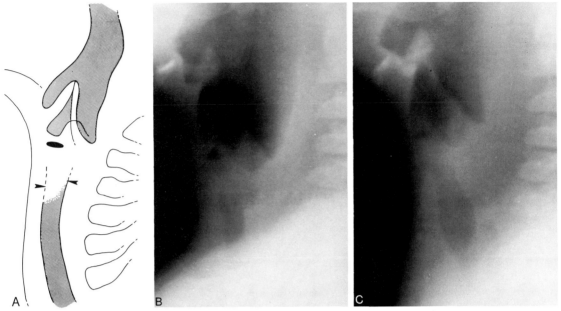

FIGURE 3–12. Croup in a 6-month-old infant with acute stridor. The line drawing (A) shows haziness of the subglottic trachea (arrowheads) consistent with the subglottic edema of croup. Lateral spot films of the upper airway made on inspiration (B) and expiration (C) show the dynamics of the subglottic obstruction. Dilatation of the hypopharynx proximal to the obstruction and constriction of the trachea distally occur during inspiration, whereas the reverse occurs during expiration.

children can be divided into two groups: those due to extrinsic tracheal compression and those due to intrinsic tracheal diseases.

EXTRINSIC TRACHEAL COMPRESSION. This type of compression may be divided into two main categories: (1) anterior compression of the cervical or intrathoracic trachea and (2) posterior compression.

The most common sources of anterior compression are cervical teratomas.[29] These midline anterior masses become very large in utero, interfere with the fetal ingestion of amniotic fluid, and cause maternal polyhydramnios. It is this progression that can lead to their diagnosis on prenatal ultrasound. At birth, infants with cervical teratomas are in serious respiratory distress, and early surgical removal is imperative. The plain film appearance of an anterior midline neck mass containing amorphous calcification, bone, and fat is typical (Fig. 3–15). An anterior cervical mass appearing in later life is more likely than not a malignant neoplasm, such as rhabdomyosarcoma or lymphoma.

The intrathoracic trachea may be compressed anteriorly by anterior mediastinal masses such as mediastinal teratomas and lymphomas (Fig. 3–16). CT[20] and, more recently, MRI[14] can detect and measure decreases in the cross-sectional areas of the trachea due to extrinsic compression (see Fig. 3–16). These values are important in the identification of children at risk of life-threatening airway compromise. It should be remembered that the normally situated, histologically normal thymus, no matter how large, does not compress the trachea or cause airway obstruction. The diseased thymus or ectopic thymus in the posterior mediastinum, however, can compromise the airway.[2]

Innominate artery compression of the trachea (anomalous innominate artery syndrome) is, at times, controversial.[1] The innominate artery normally passes anterior to the trachea and, in so doing, can cause an indentation on its anterior

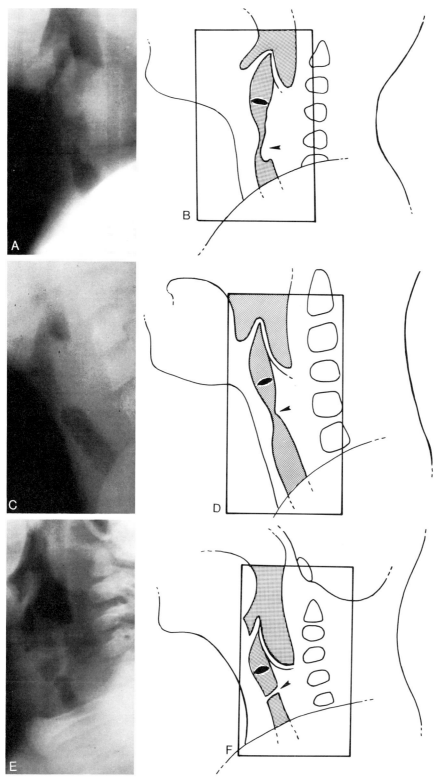

FIGURE 3–13. Subglottic stenosis in three infants following prolonged endotracheal intubation. The radiograph (*A*) and corresponding line drawing (*B*) demonstrate an irregular narrowing of the subglottic trachea due to mounds of granulation tissue (arrowhead). The radiograph (*C*) and corresponding line drawing (*D*) show a concentric stenosis in the subglottic trachea (arrowhead). The radiograph (*E*) and corresponding line drawing (*F*) show a cicatricial band or web (arrowhead) in the same area. (*A*, *C*, and *E* reprinted with permission from Macpherson RI, Leithiser RE: Upper airway obstruction in children: An update. Radiographics 5:339–376, 1985.)

45

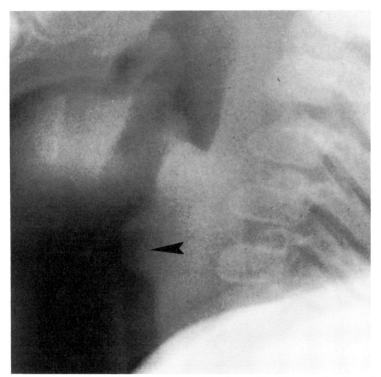

FIGURE 3–14. Subglottic mucocele in a 6-month-old infant with a history of prolonged endotracheal intubation. The lateral view of the airway shows a smooth, rounded mass in the subglottic trachea (arrowhead). At endoscopy, this was a mucus-filled cyst.

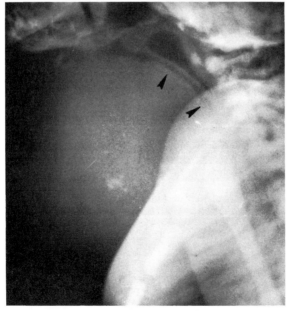

FIGURE 3–15. Cervical teratoma in a newborn male with respiratory distress. The lateral view of the neck shows a large, calcium-containing mass anterior to and compressing the trachea (arrowheads). This is a surgical emergency. (Reprinted with permission from Macpherson RI, Leithiser RE: Upper airway obstruction in children: An update. Radiographics 5:339–376, 1985.)

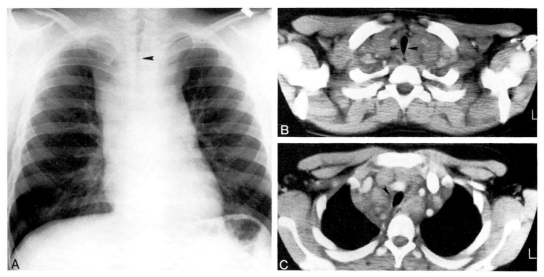

FIGURE 3–16. Mediastinal Hodgkin's disease in a 12-year-old male with respiratory distress. The frontal chest radiograph (A) shows the large anterior and superior mediastinal mass compressing the trachea (arrowhead). CT sections at the thoracic inlet (B) and superior mediastinal (C) levels show lateral and anterior compression of the trachea by the mass (arrowheads).

aspect. This indentation can be seen in asymptomatic children[37] as well as in children with stridor in whom innominate artery compression of the trachea has been implicated (Fig. 3–17). The pulsatile indentation caused by the "anomalous innominate" can be seen at endoscopy and fluoroscopy. Surgical suspension of the innominate artery anteriorly to the manubrium has brought relief of symptoms in these children. It is difficult for the radiologist to differentiate between the normal innominate indentation of the trachea and that caused by "anomalous innominate artery syndrome." (Editor's note: Angiography may demonstrate an origin for the artery that, because it is located farther along the arch, affords more contact with the trachea.)

Infants who have had repair of esophageal atresia can present with apneic spells associated with feeding.[13] In these children, the distending proximal esophagus may displace the trachea anteriorly and compress it against a normal innominate artery (Fig. 3–18). There is no doubt, in this situation, that the innominate artery acts as a cause of airway obstruction.

Compression of the posterior aspect of the trachea may be produced by vascular anomalies,[35] such as rings and slings. Although anomalies of the aortic arch are common, the majority are asymptomatic and remain undetected. Stridor, cyanotic attacks, recurrent respiratory infections, and dysphagia during the first year of life are symptoms suggestive of a possible aortic arch anomaly or "vascular ring."

There are many varieties of vascular rings, some of which are complete, or "closed," and others of which are incomplete, or "open." Double aortic arch (Fig. 3–19) and right aortic arch are the most common complete vascular rings, and the anomalous right subclavian artery is the most prevalent incomplete vascular ring. The demonstration, by esophagography, of a persistent indentation on the posterior aspect of the esophagus (Fig. 3–19A) is highly suggestive of a vascular ring. Aortography (Fig. 3–19B) and, recently, CT[20] and MRI[14] have been used to delineate the exact nature of the anomaly.

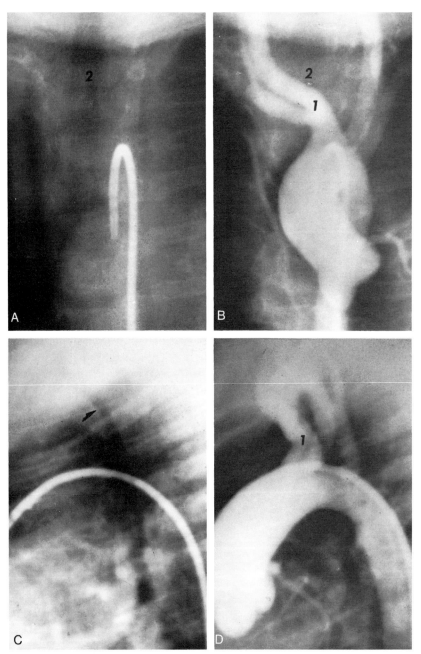

FIGURE 3–17. Innominate artery syndrome in an infant with stridor. The relationship of the innominate artery to the trachea is shown by aortography. On the AP view, before (*A*) and during (*B*) contrast injection, and on the lateral views, before (*C*) and during (*D*) injection, the branching innominate artery (*1*) passes in front of the trachea (*2*). Note the indentation on the anterior aspect of the trachea (arrowhead) attributed to innominate artery compression. (Reprinted with permission from Macpherson RI, Leithiser RE: Upper airway obstruction in children: An update. Radiographics 5:339–376, 1985.)

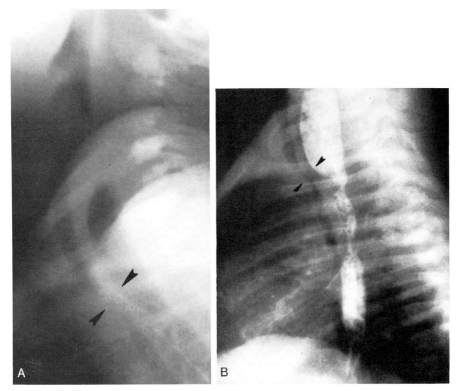

FIGURE 3–18. Innominate artery compression of the trachea in a 6-week-old infant following repair of esophageal atresia. The compression of the trachea between the dilated proximal esophagus and the innominate artery can be appreciated on the lateral view of the airway (A), wherein the proximal portion is distended with air (arrowheads), and the esophagogram (B), wherein it is visualized with barium (arrowheads). (Reprinted with permission from Macpherson RI, Leithiser RE: Upper airway obstruction in children: An update. Radiographics 5:339–376, 1985.)

A pulmonary artery sling[5] is an unusual vascular anomaly in which the left pulmonary artery arises from the right pulmonary artery and passes between the trachea and the esophagus en route to the left lung (Fig. 3–20). In so doing, the pulmonary artery can compress the trachea and, as a result, cause respiratory distress in infants. Pulmonary artery sling is often associated with long-segment, congenital tracheal stenosis due to "complete tracheal rings" (Fig. 3–21). This combination, called the "ring-sling complex," presents a more serious and difficult management problem than does the pulmonary artery sling alone.

The diagnosis of pulmonary artery sling can be suspected on chest radiography (see Fig. 6–7A) and confirmed by esophagography (see Fig. 3–20A) and angiography (see Fig. 3–20C). An associated tracheal anomaly can be suspected on the basis of airway studies and, if necessary, confirmed by xerography (see Fig. 3–21A) or, better still, tracheography (see Figs. 3–20B and 3–21B).

In addition to pulmonary artery sling, bronchogenic cysts (Fig. 3–22), ectopic thyroid, neurofibromatosis, mediastinal abscesses, and other rare abnormalities such as a ductus arteriosus sling can be found between the trachea and the esophagus. Bronchogenic cysts may be found in a variety of locations within the chest and may have a number of different clinical presentations. These cysts should be the first consideration, however, when one discovers a mass resting

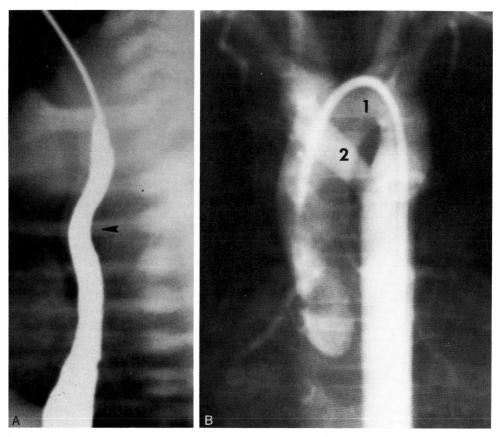

FIGURE 3–19. Vascular ring in an infant with stridor. An esophagogram (*A*) shows an indentation on the posterior aspect of the esophagus (arrowhead) consistent with a vascular ring. An aortogram (*B*) can be used to demonstrate the type of vascular ring, in this case, a double aortic arch. The ascending aorta divides into a left arch (*1*) that passes in front of the trachea and the esophagus and a right arch (*2*) that passes behind, in doing so, compressing the posterior aspect of the esophagus. (*A* reprinted with permission from Macpherson RI, Leithiser RE: Upper airway obstruction in children: An update. Radiographics 5:339–376, 1985.)

between the trachea and the esophagus in an infant with respiratory distress (Fig. 3–22*B*). CT (Fig. 3–22*C*) can be used to confirm the diagnosis. It must be remembered, however, that the fluid in bronchogenic cysts may have a high mucoid content; as such, they may have attenuation values on CT above those usually considered pathognomonic of a cyst.

An intraesophageal foreign body can also compress the trachea posteriorly.[33] A foreign body lodged in the esophagus can compress the trachea directly (Fig. 3–23), through esophageal distension, or by causing paraesophageal, soft tissue swelling. Often, an esophageal stricture, such as a postoperative esophageal atresia repair, will predispose a child to foreign body impaction. If a child with a history of esophageal stricture presents with acute stridor following ingestion of solid food, the probability of a foreign body lodged above the stricture should be considered.

INTRINSIC TRACHEAL DISEASES. The intrinsic tracheal diseases that cause respiratory obstruction in children are generally the most difficult lesions to manage. One such lesion, congenital tracheal stenosis (Fig. 3–24),[28] is a rare, life-threatening anomaly seen in three forms: a generalized tracheal hypoplasia; a funnellike, distal tracheal narrowing; and segmental stenosis. Often, the nor-

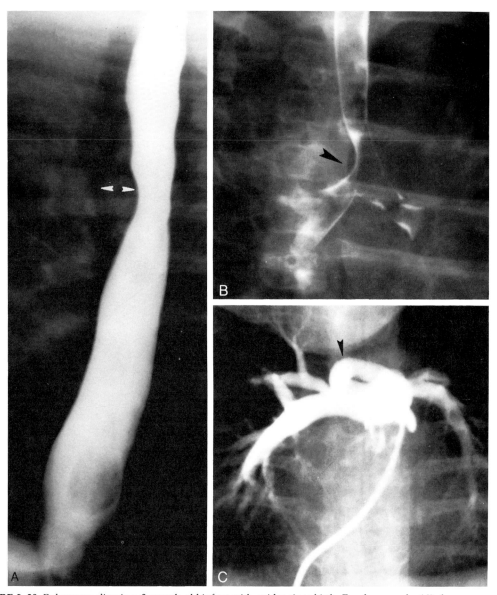

FIGURE 3–20. Pulmonary sling in a 3-month-old infant with stridor since birth. Esophagography (*A*) shows a mass separating the air-filled trachea from the barium-filled esophagus (arrowheads). Tracheography (*B*) shows the indentation on the right side of the trachea just above the carina on its posterolateral aspect (arrowhead). Pulmonary angiography (*C*) shows the anomalous left pulmonary artery (arrowhead) arising from the right pulmonary artery, to the right of the trachea, passing behind it en route to the left lung. (Courtesy of Dr. Joe Jackson, Driscoll Foundation Children's Hospital, Corpus Christi, Texas.)

mally horseshoe-shaped cartilaginous rings completely encircle the trachea and, in so doing, form complete tracheal rings. This tracheal anomaly is frequently associated with a pulmonary artery sling, a combination designated the "ring-sling complex." With or without pulmonary sling, however, congenital tracheal stenosis presents a difficult management problem. Fortunately, in recent years, newer surgical techniques have provided an improved prognosis in these children.

The incidence of acquired tracheal stenosis (Fig. 3–25) has increased with the widespread use of tracheal intubation for ventilatory assistance.[40] Both endotra-

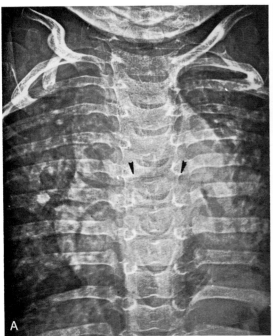

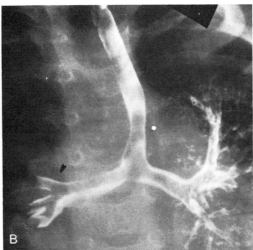

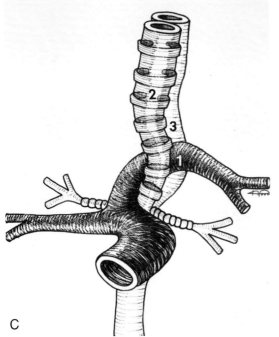

FIGURE 3–21. Pulmonary sling with complete tracheal rings in a 3-week-old infant with respiratory distress since birth. Frontal xerography of the chest (A) shows a deviation of the trachea to the left and a horizontal orientation of the main bronchi or the "inverted T appearance" (arrowheads). Tracheography (B) shows the tracheal deviation, inverted T appearance, and typical distal take-off of the right upper lobe bronchus (arrowhead). The line drawing (C) puts all the components together: the left pulmonary artery (1), the trachea (2) with its complete rings, and the esophagus (3), in the "ring-sling complex." (Reprinted with permission from Macpherson RI, Leithiser RE: Upper airway obstruction in children: An update. Radiographics 5:339–376, 1985.)

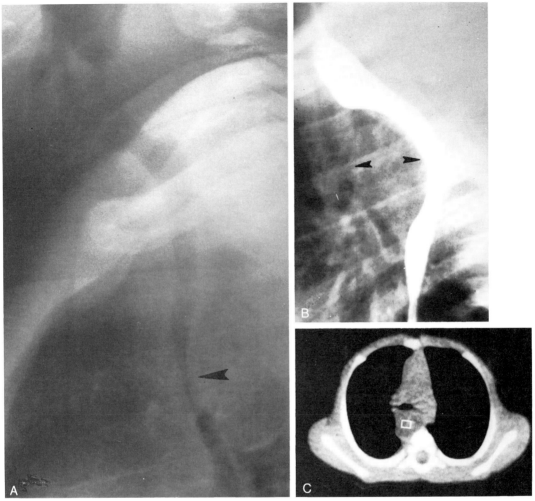

FIGURE 3–22. Bronchogenic cyst in a 6-week-old infant with respiratory distress since birth. The lateral airway film (*A*) shows a posterior impression on the trachea just above the carina (arrowhead). An esophagogram (*B*) shows a mass between the trachea and esophagus (arrowheads). CT (*C*) demonstrates a relatively high-density, presumably mucus-containing cyst (cursor) behind the trachea. A diagnosis of bronchogenic cyst was confirmed at surgery. (Reprinted with permission from Macpherson RI, Leithiser RE: Upper airway obstruction in children: An update. Radiographics 5:339–376, 1985.)

cheal and tracheostomy tubes are to blame for this problem. The symptoms, which appear within 2 months of extubation, vary from dyspnea on exertion to extreme dyspnea with stridor. The initial reaction to tracheal intubation is granuloma formation (Fig. 3–26), which is followed by mucosal ulceration, cartilage destruction (acquired tracheomalacia), and eventual scar formation with stenosis. Tracheal stenosis can also be acquired as a result of direct trauma to the trachea (Fig. 3–27), tracheal tumors (Fig. 3–28), and infections.

Tracheal tumors (see Fig. 3–28), the majority of which are benign, are rare causes of airway obstruction in children.[41] Squamous cell papillomas, fibromas, and hemangiomas are most commonly seen. Papillomas may arise as a progression of laryngeal papillomatosis or occur separately (Fig. 3–28*A*). Fibromas (Fig. 3–28*B*) are slow growing, intramural lesions and are usually asymptomatic during childhood. Tracheal hemangiomas, although commonly found in the

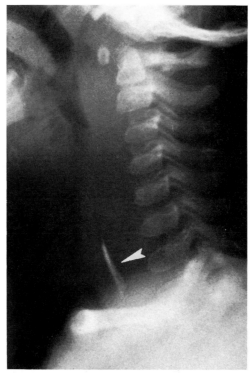

FIGURE 3–23. Esophageal foreign body in a 3-year-old male with acute stridor. The lateral view of the upper airway shows a radiopaque foreign body (pork chop bone) in the cervical esophagus at the thoracic inlet (arrowhead), compressing the trachea from behind. The symptoms were relieved by endoscopic removal of the foreign body. (Reprinted with permission from Macpherson RI, Leithiser RE: Upper airway obstruction in children: An update. Radiographics 5:339–376, 1985.)

subglottic region, can occur in the more distal portions of the trachea and produce symptoms of respiratory distress in children.

Endotracheal foreign bodies (Fig. 3–29) are much less common than their endobronchial counterparts[42] and most often lodge in the subglottic trachea, the narrowest part of the child's airway.

Tracheomalacia[6] is characterized by abnormal tracheal collapse secondary to inadequacy of tracheal cartilage, the latter due either to congenital immaturity (primary tracheomalacia) or cartilaginous degeneration (secondary tracheomalacia) following an inflammatory process, extrinsic pressure, bronchial neoplasms, or tracheoesophageal fistula. Primary tracheomalacia is characterized by an expiratory, often self-limiting "stridor" in infancy (Fig. 3–30). It must be remembered, however, that the normal trachea will show some variation in caliber during respiration; as such, it can be difficult to differentiate between mild tracheomalacia and a normal variation.

Mainstem Bronchi

The mainstem bronchi comprise the last segment of the upper airway. Congenital causes of obstruction in this area are usually symptomatic in infancy and can be divided into two main groups: those that cause extrinsic compression of the bronchus and those that originate in the bronchial wall itself.

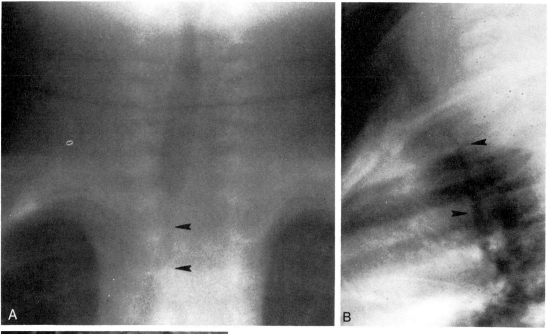

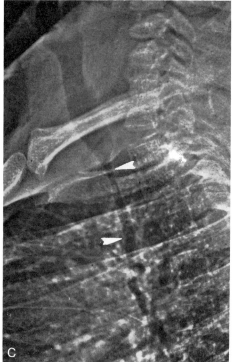

FIGURE 3–24. Congenital tracheal stenosis in a newborn with respiratory distress. On the frontal magnification view of the airway (*A*), a long segmental stenosis of the distal trachea is seen (arrowheads). The lateral magnification view (*B*) and xerography (*C*) show the same lesion beginning below the thoracic inlet and extending to the carina (arrowheads). Note the enhanced visibility of this complete ring, congenital tracheal stenosis on xerography. (Reprinted with permission from Macpherson RI, Leithiser RE: Upper airway obstruction in children: An update. Radiographics 5:339–376, 1985.)

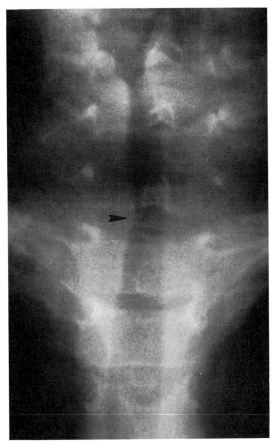

FIGURE 3–25. Acquired tracheal stenosis in a 13-year-old female who was intubated during infancy. Thereafter, she had 40 hospital admissions for the treatment of a recurrent localized stenosis in the cervical portion of the trachea (arrowhead). (Reprinted with permission from Macpherson RI, Leithiser RE: Upper airway obstruction in children: An update. Radiographics 5:339–376, 1985.)

Pulmonary vascular sling can cause extrinsic compression, usually of the right mainstem bronchus, as the left pulmonary artery swings around the trachea to pass between the trachea and the esophagus en route to the left lung (see Fig. 3–20). Bronchogenic cysts[11] (Fig. 3–31), which constitute 5% of all mediastinal masses in children, can also compress mainstem bronchi, usually the left. Mediastinal bronchogenic cysts can have a subcarinal location, and, although they are often small (less than 2 cm in diameter) and imperceptible on plain chest radiographs, they are capable of causing significant bronchial obstruction. Esophagography is useful in demonstrating the presence of these often subtle masses (Fig. 3–31B). CT can also be used to identify the site, size, and nature of the lesions.[27] Note that bronchogenic cysts can be deceptively dense owing to their high mucoid content and that calcium is occasionally found in their walls and contents.

The congenital obstructing lesions that originate in the bronchial wall itself include bronchial atresia, bronchial stenosis, bronchial web, and bronchomalacia. Each of these congenital abnormalities, extrinsic and intramural, can affect the adjacent lung in four ways. The most common means is through obstructive overinflation (congenital lobar emphysema), wherein a check-valve type of obstruction causes the affected lung to become progressively overinflated. As a

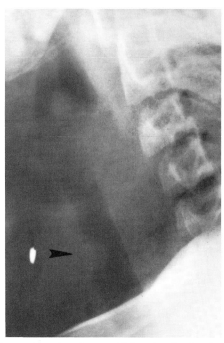

FIGURE 3–26. Tracheal granuloma in a 3-year-old female who developed respiratory distress following removal of a tracheostomy tube. On the lateral view of the upper airway, a polypoid filling defect is seen in the trachea at the tracheostomy site (arrowhead; opposite the metal skin clip). A granuloma was removed at endoscopy, and the symptoms were relieved. (Reprinted with permission from Macpherson RI, Leithiser RE: Upper airway obstruction in children: An update. Radiographics 5:339–376, 1985.)

result, the mediastinum is moved away from the affected side and the normal lobes are compromised. The second way is through obstructive atelectasis, wherein complete bronchial obstruction causes the affected lung to undergo absorption collapse. Consequently, displacement of the mediastinum toward the affected side occurs. A third appearance is that of recurrent pneumonia proximal to the obstruction. The final presentation, seen only in the newborn, is that of an opaque, overdistended lung (Fig. 3–31A).[17] This phenomenon occurs when, owing to an obstruction, the normal fetal lung fluid is trapped within the lung and overdistends it.

The acquired causes of bronchial obstruction in children can be divided into three subgroups (extrinsic, intramural, and intraluminal), all of which are capable of producing obstructive overinflation. Extrinsic obstruction of the bronchi can be acquired as a result of peribronchial lymphadenopathy secondary to infections such as primary tuberculosis, histoplasmosis, infectious mononucleosis, or lymphoma. Intramural bronchial obstruction can be caused by such things as endobronchial tuberculosis, granulation tissue secondary to intubation, or peripheral seeding of laryngeal papillomatosis.

Aspirated foreign bodies, which are the most common of all bronchial obstructions, head the list of intraluminal causes of airway obstruction in children. Approximately 80% of all affected children are less than 3 years of age; the aspirated foreign body is food or food products 70% of the time, with peanuts comprising 40% of the entire group.[42] The anatomic sites within the tracheobronchial tree where foreign bodies are found at the time of endoscopy are, in decreasing order of frequency, the right mainstem bronchus (34%), the left mainstem bronchus (31%), the right bronchus intermedius (11%), the right

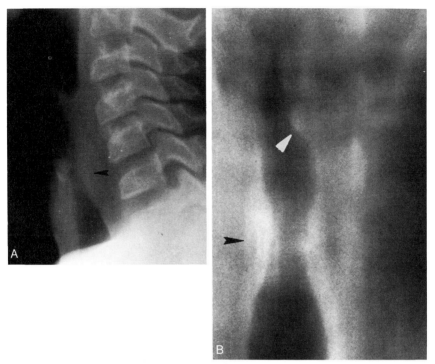

FIGURE 3-27. Traumatic tracheal stricture in a teen-aged male who ruptured his trachea at 8 years of age from a clothesline injury. The lateral view of the airway (*A*) shows a calcifying stricture in the cervical portion of the trachea (arrowhead). Linear tomography in the frontal plane (*B*) shows the circumferential nature of the lesion (black arrowhead) and a subglottic stenosis (white arrowhead) from the prolonged intubation at time of injury. (Reprinted with permission from Macpherson RI, Leithiser RE: Upper airway obstruction in children: An update. Radiographics 5:339–376, 1985.)

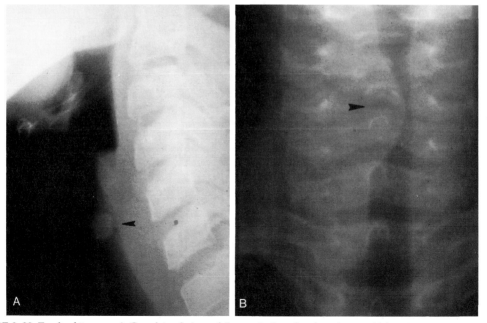

FIGURE 3-28. Tracheal tumors. *A,* On a lateral view of the cervical trachea in a 6-year-old female with stridor, an intraluminal polypoid lesion (arrowhead) is seen. A squamous papilloma was removed by endoscopy. *B,* On the frontal view of the cervical trachea in a 15-year-old female with chronic stridor, an intramural mass is seen (arrowhead). An intramural fibroma was removed at surgery. (Reprinted with permission from Macpherson RI, Leithiser RE: Upper airway obstruction in children: An update. Radiographics 5:339–376, 1985.)

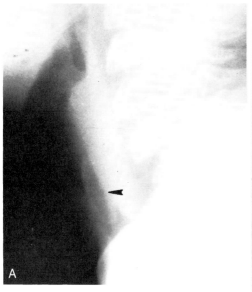

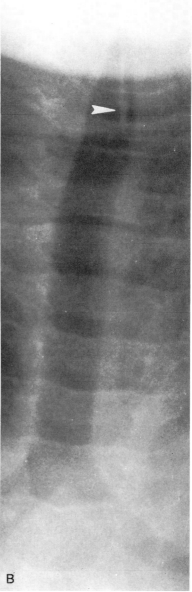

FIGURE 3–29. Endotracheal foreign bodies. *A*, The lateral view of the upper airway in a 3-year-old female with acute stridor shows an intraluminal filling defect (arrowhead). At endoscopy, a sunflower seed husk was removed. *B*, A frontal view of the airway in a 1-year-old female with stridor shows a vertical linear filling defect (arrowhead) in the subglottic trachea. At endoscopy, a piece of a leaf was removed. (*A* reprinted with permission from Macpherson RI, Leithiser RE: Upper airway obstruction in children: An update. Radiographics 5:339–376, 1985.)

lower lobe bronchus (9%), the left lower lobe bronchus (8%), the trachea (4%), and bilaterally (4%).[42]

Because only 6% of all aspirated foreign bodies are radiopaque, we must rely, in most instances, on secondary changes in the lungs to make a radiologic diagnosis, which, incidentally, can be achieved in only 70% of the cases. Negative radiologic studies, therefore, cannot be used to exclude the diagnosis. The most common positive finding is obstructive overinflation due to the check-valve effect created by the foreign body in the bronchus (Fig. 3–32). In these cases, the posteroanterior (PA) view of the chest made in deep inspiration may appear normal or exhibit some hyperlucency with or without overdistension of the affected lung. At fluoroscopy or on films made during expiration, any air trapping will be amplified, as air can escape the normal lung but not the obstructed

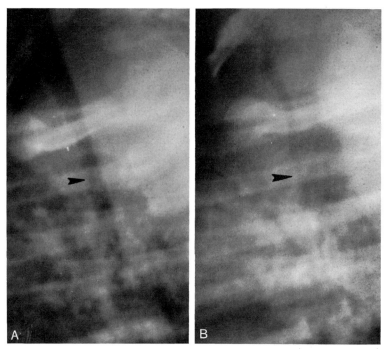

FIGURE 3-30. Tracheomalacia in a 3-week-old infant with noisy breathing. The lateral fluoroscopic spot films show the AP diameter of the thoracic trachea (arrowheads) to be normal during inspiration (*A*), but markedly narrowed during expiration (*B*). This narrowing is considered in excess of normal and is consistent with primary tracheomalacia. (Reprinted with permission from Macpherson RI, Leithiser RE: Upper airway obstruction in children: An update. Radiographics 5:339–376, 1985.)

one. Thus, the heart and mediastinum will shift away from the affected side during expiration. This phenomenon is the hallmark of check-valve obstruction, regardless of the etiology, and can be witnessed dynamically at fluoroscopy, our diagnostic method of choice.

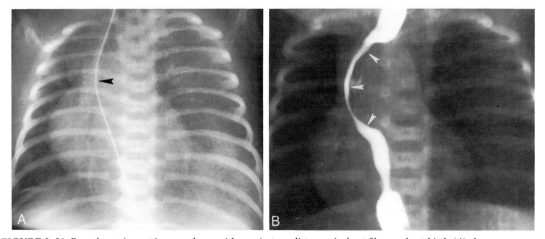

FIGURE 3-31. Bronchogenic cyst in a newborn with respiratory distress. A chest film made at birth (*A*) shows an opaque overdistended left lung displacing the mediastinum to the right. This suggests a partial obstruction of the left main bronchus with retention of lung fluid distally. The marked displacement of the esophagus, as indicated by the nasogastric tube (arrowhead), suggests a mediastinal mass. An esophagogram (*B*) outlines the mediastinal mass (arrowheads), which at surgery was a bronchogenic cyst.

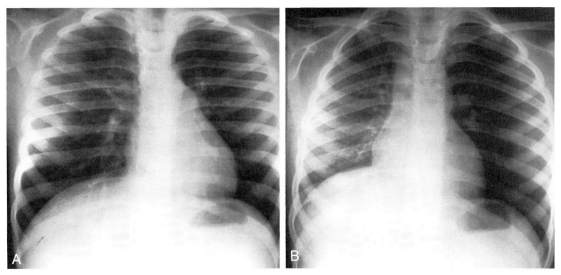

FIGURE 3–32. Intrabronchial foreign body in a 3-year-old child with an acute onset of wheezing. A frontal chest film made on inspiration (*A*) shows the left lung to be slightly hyperlucent. This is subtle evidence of check-valve obstruction. On expiration (*B*), the egress of air from the left lung is impeded and it stays inflated, whereas the right lung deflates. As a consequence, the mediastinum shifts away from the affected side during expiration, confirming the suspicion of a check-valve obstruction in the left main bronchus. In children, this is usually a nonopaque foreign body.

Lateral decubitus projections of the chest have been used in the diagnosis of check-valve obstruction due to intrabronchial foreign bodies. Ordinarily, when a child is lying on his side, the dependent lung tends to be underaerated. When there is a check-valve obstruction, however, the dependent lung remains well inflated. Advocates of lateral decubitus chest projections claim the method is more reliable than inspiration-expiration chest films or fluoroscopy. In our limited experience, however, we have found it to be equivocal and have continued to rely on fluoroscopy for this purpose.

Other findings on chest film suggestive of the possibility of an intrabronchial foreign body are atelectasis of a lobe or lung and persistent lobar pneumonia (Fig. 3–33). The longer a foreign body is retained within the airway, the greater

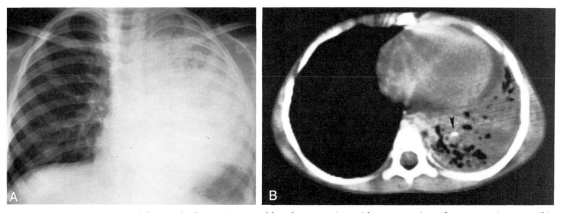

FIGURE 3–33. Intrabronchial foreign body in a 1-year-old male presenting with pneumonia and unresponsive to antibiotics. A plain chest radiograph (*A*) shows a relatively small, opaque left lung containing perceptible air-filled bronchi. CT section (*B*) shows a small oval density (arrowhead) within the consolidated, partially collapsed left lung. A piece of chicken bone was removed by endoscopy, and the infection cleared rapidly.

the likelihood of these complications.[42] In such instances, CT can be used to identify intrabronchial foreign bodies imperceptible even at bronchoscopy (see Fig. 3–33).

After reviewing the many causes of airway obstruction in children and the current status of the radiologic technology available to investigate them, one has to conclude that the radiology department plays, and will continue to play, a major role in the management of children with this problem.

REFERENCES

1. Ardito JM, Ossoff RH, Tucker GF, Deleon SY: Innominate artery compression of the trachea with reflex apnea. Ann Otol Rhinol Laryngol 89:410–415, 1980
2. Bar-Ziv J, Barki Y, Itzchak Y, Mares AJ: Posterior mediastinal accessory thymus. Pediatr Radiol 14:165–167, 1984
3. Benjamin B: Congenital laryngeal webs. Ann Otol Rhinol Laryngol 92:317–326, 1983
4. Benjamin B, Carter P: Congenital hemangioma. Ann Otol Rhinol Laryngol 92:448–455, 1983
5. Berdon WE, Baker D, Wung J, et al: Complete cartilage-ring tracheal stenosis associated with anomalous left pulmonary artery: The ring-sling complex. Radiology 152:57–64, 1984
6. Cogbill TH, Moore FA, Accurso FJ, Lilly JR: Primary tracheomalacia. Ann Thorac Surg 35:538–541, 1983
7. Cohen SR, Geller KA, Seltzer S, Thompson JW: Papilloma of the larynx and tracheobronchial tree in children: A retrospective study. Ann Otol Rhinol Laryngol 89:497–503, 1980
8. Currarino G, Williams B: Lateral inspiration and expiration radiographs of the neck in children with laryngotracheitis (croup). Radiology 145:365–366, 1982
9. Dagin R, Leiberman A, Strauss R, et al: Subglottic mucocele in an infant. Pediatr Radiol 8:119–121, 1979
10. Dunbar JS: Upper respiratory tract obstruction in infants and children. AJR 109:225–246, 1970
11. Eraklis AJ, Griscom NT, McGovern JB: Bronchogenic cysts of the mediastinum in infancy. N Engl J Med 281:1150–1155, 1969
12. Fernback S, Brouillette RT, Riggs TW, Hunt CE: Radiologic evaluation of adenoids and tonsils in children with obstructive sleep apnea: Plain films and fluoroscopy. Pediatr Radiol 13:258–265, 1983
13. Filler RM, Rossello PJ, Lebowitz RL: Life threatening anoxic spells caused by tracheal compression after repair of esophageal atresia: Correction by surgery. J Pediatr Surg 11:739–746, 1976
14. Fletcher BD, Dearborn DG, Mulopulos GP: MR imaging in infants with airway obstruction: Preliminary observations. Radiology 160:245–249, 1986
15. Frech RS, McAlister WH: Teratoma of the nasopharynx producing depression of the posterior hard palate. J Can Assoc Radiol 20:204–205, 1969
16. Fujioka M, Young LW, Girdany BR: Radiographic evaluation of adenoidal size in children: Adenoidal nasopharyngeal ratio. AJR 133:401–404, 1979
17. Griscom NT, Harris GBC, Wohl MEB, Vawter GF, Eraklis AJ: Fluid filled lung due to airway obstruction in the newborn. Pediatrics 43:383–390, 1969
18. Heller RM, Kirchner SG, O'Neil JA: Xeroradiographic evaluation of obstructive lesions of the larynx and trachea. J Pediatr Surg 16:691–733, 1981
19. Joseph PM, Berdon WE, Baker DH, et al: Upper airway obstruction in infants and small children: Improved radiographic diagnosis by combining filtration, high kilovoltage and magnification. Radiology 121:148, 1976
20. Kirks DR, Fram EK, Vock P, Effman EL: Tracheal compression by mediastinal masses in children: CT evaluation. AJR 141:647–651, 1983
21. Lind MG, Lindell BPW: Tonsillar hyperplasia in children: A cause of obstructive sleep apneas, CO_2 retention and retarded growth. Arch Otolaryngol 108:650–654, 1982
22. Macpherson RI, Leithiser RE: Upper airway obstruction in children: An update. Radiographics 5:339–376, 1985
23. Marshak G, Grundfast KM: Subglottic stenosis. Pediatr Clin North Am 28:941–948, 1981
24. McCook TA, Felman AH: Retropharyngeal masses in infants and children. Am J Dis Child 133:41–43, 1979
25. McCook TA, Kirks DR: Epiglottic enlargement in infants and children: Another radiologic look. Pediatr Radiol 12:227–234, 1982
26. Miller EN, Norman D: The role of computed tomography in the evaluation of neck masses. Radiology 133:144–149, 1979
27. Nakata H, Nakayama C, Kimoto T, et al: Computed tomography of the mediastinal bronchogenic cysts. J Comput Assist Tomogr 6:733–738, 1982
28. Nakayama DK, Harrison MR, deLorimier AA, et al: Reconstructive surgery for obstructing lesions of the intrathoracic trachea in infants and small children. J Pediatr Surg 17:854–868, 1982

29. Patel RB, Gibson JY, D'Cruz CA, Burkhalter JL: Sonographic diagnosis of cervical teratoma in utero. AJR 139:1220–1222, 1982
30. Pounds LA: Neck masses of congenital origin. Pediatr Clin North Am 28:841–844, 1981
31. Shackelford GD, McAlister WH: Congenital laryngeal cyst. AJR 114:289–292, 1972
32. Siegel MJ, Nadel SN, Glazer HS, et al: Mediastinal lesions in childhood: Comparison of CT and MR. Radiology 160:241–244, 1986
33. Smith PC, Swischuk LE, Fagan CJ: An elusive and often unsuspected cause of stridor or pneumonia (the esophageal foreign body). AJR 122:178–185, 1974
34. Smith RJ, Catlin FI: Congenital anomalies of the larynx. Am J Dis Child 138:35–39, 1984
35. Smith RJ, Smith MC, Glossup P, et al: Congenital vascular anomalies causing tracheoesophageal compression. Arch Otolaryngol 110:82–87, 1984
36. Som PM, Cohen BA, Sacher M, et al: The angiomatous polyp and the angiofibroma: Two different lesions. Radiology 144:329–334, 1982
37. Swischuk LE: Anterior tracheal indentation in infancy and early childhood: Normal or abnormal? AJR 112:12–17, 1971
38. Swischuk LE, Smith PC, Fagan CJ: Abnormalities of the pharynx and larynx in childhood. Semin Roentgenol 9:283–300, 1974
39. Theogaraj SD, Hoehn JG, Hagan KF: Practical management of congenital choanal atresia. Plast Reconstr Surg 72:634–640, 1983
40. Weber AL, Grillo HC: Tracheal stenosis: An analysis of 151 cases. Radiol Clin North Am 16:291–308, 1978
41. Weber AL, Grillo HC: Tracheal tumors: A radiological, clinical and pathological evaluation of 84 cases. Radiol Clin North Am 16:227–246, 1978
42. Wiseman NE: The diagnosis of foreign body aspiration in childhood. J Pediatr Surg 19:531–535, 1984

chapter 4

Medical Diseases of the Airway: A Surgeon's Role

H. Biemann Othersen, Jr., M.D.

Respiratory problems are common in the pediatric practice and are typically well handled by pediatricians. The pediatrician may, however, need help in establishing a difficult airway. Similarly, emergency room physicians often require surgical consultation when small children experience airway distress. Given this interplay among pediatricians, emergency room physicians, and surgeons, it is imperative that medical practitioners within a community establish a local protocol for the management of children with airway problems. Once devised, the protocol should be promulgated and followed (Figs. 4–1 and 4–2).

The examining pediatrician is usually able to differentiate between problems in the upper airway—the larynx and trachea—and those in the bronchi and bronchioles. In addition to foreign body obstruction of the airway, there are four medical conditions that cause upper airway distress: spasmodic croup, laryngotracheobronchitis, bacterial tracheitis, and epiglottitis. There is a current tendency to group all of these conditions under the term "croup syndrome."[10] We, however, single out epiglottitis and prefer to use the term "croup" to refer only to spasmodic croup, laryngotracheobronchitis, and bacterial tracheitis. A careful history and physical examination are usually the best means by which to differentiate these processes.[7]

PROCEDURE

The surgeon should insist that the pediatrician notify him or her as soon as a child with severe respiratory distress is seen. Depending on the child's condition, emergency endoscopy in the operating room in a controlled environment may prove necessary.

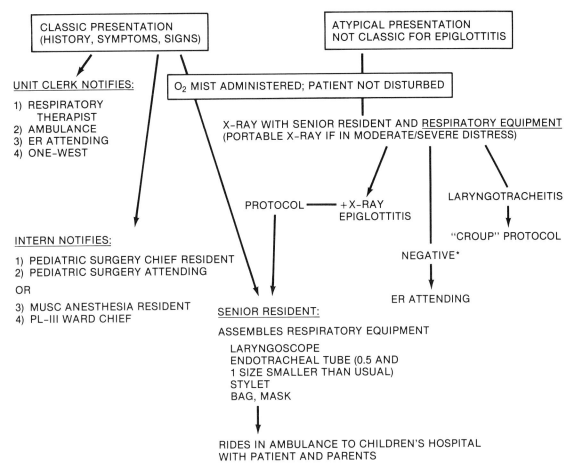

FIGURE 4-1. Medical University of South Carolina Children's Hospital emergency room protocol for epiglottitis management.

Unless the situation is desperate and the child is exchanging no air at all, it may be unwise to attempt examination of the epiglottis or intubation in the emergency room. The child's violent struggles and cries may precipitate complete airway obstruction when the supraglottic structures are already edematous and inflamed. The child who is obviously severely compromised and in whom epiglottic or supraglottic edema exists should be brought immediately to the operating area where he or she can be seen by an anesthesiologist and a surgeon. There, the anesthesiologist will attempt intubation; if intubation is unsuccessful, the surgeon will introduce the rigid bronchoscope. In the rare instance that a small endotracheal tube or bronchoscope cannot be introduced, immediate tracheostomy should be performed.

Spasmodic Croup

Patients with spasmodic croup are well managed by pediatricians and family physicians; as a result, the surgeon seldom sees these patients. The child with spasmodic croup is typically between 1 and 3 years of age and presents with a

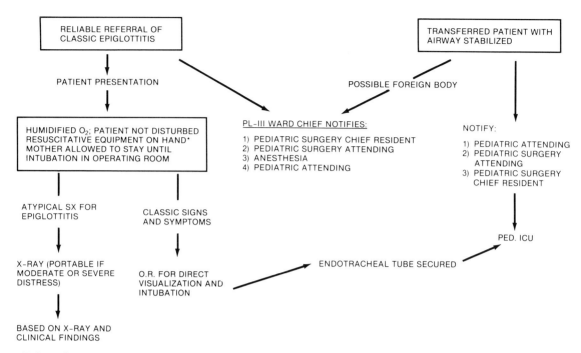

FIGURE 4-2. Direct referral, Medical University of South Carolina Children's Hospital emergency protocol for epiglottitis management.

sudden onset of symptoms, the first of which is frequently a harsh, barking cough. Coughing and inspiratory stridor usually occur at night and often awaken the child from sleep. There is rarely any antecedent infection or respiratory illness, and the child is usually not cyanotic. Because this condition rapidly responds to humidification of inspired air, hospitalization is rarely necessary. Note that spasmodic croup is the most likely diagnosis if the affected child was awakened from sleep and developed croup without any antecedent symptoms. If, however, the child had been playing with small toys when the symptoms appeared, foreign body aspiration should be suspected, and endoscopy is indicated.

Laryngotracheobronchitis

Laryngotracheobronchitis is the condition usually called "croup." It is seen most frequently in children from 3 months to 3 years of age, with a peak incidence occurring during the 2nd year of life. The condition usually develops during the winter season, and its etiology almost always consists of a viral infection with a history of an antecedent respiratory infection of gradual onset. Typically, a mild cough will progress to a harsh cough, which will then gradually lead to inspiratory stridor and dyspnea. The child with laryngotracheobronchitis will commonly have an elevated temperature.

Hospital admission is usually advisable for the child with laryngotracheobronchitis. The hospitalized patient can be observed with pulse oximetry,[6] humidification of inspired air, and racemic epinephrine (0.25 to 0.5 ml diluted to 2 ml of saline) delivered by nebulization. If there is no immediate improvement or if cyanosis is present, the child should be taken directly to the operating room for evaluation and treatment by both an anesthesiologist and a surgeon.

Mild cases of laryngotracheobronchitis with moderate edema usually respond to racemic epinephrine inhalations. More advanced edema and airway obstruction may require judicious endotracheal intubation. If the endotracheal tube is not too tight and it is felt that the edema may subside within 24 to 48 hours, intubation should be continued with immediate administration of intravenous steroids (dexamethasone 0.8 mg/kg/day divided and given every 6 hours). If, however, the edema is severe, an airway should be established with an endotracheal tube or bronchoscope and a tracheostomy performed. These patients are usually decannulated as soon as the edema has subsided.

Bacterial Tracheitis

Often referred to as membranous laryngotracheobronchitis, bacterial tracheitis is an acute, nonviral, infectious disease. Not as common as viral croup and seen in children of any age, bacterial tracheitis is an infection caused by virulent bacteria such as *Staphylococcus aureus.* This bacterial infection may be superimposed on a viral laryngotracheobronchitis. Affected children present with a clinical picture similar to that of croup. Unlike croup, however, they rapidly develop severe upper airway obstruction and a high fever. Children with bacterial tracheitis also may have a very toxic appearance, and endoscopy often shows mucopurulent secretions.

Diagnosis of bacterial tracheitis is made by endoscopy and tracheal cultures. As in cases of laryngotracheobronchitis, however, if there is extensive inflammatory disease of the larynx and upper trachea, an endotracheal tube should be inserted for an airway and a temporary tracheostomy performed.

Epiglottitis

Epiglottitis is usually seen in, but is not limited to, young children between the ages of 2 and 6. Patients with epiglottitis, a condition often abrupt in onset, complain of a sore throat and dysphagia. Their temperature is usually high, their speech may be slurred, and drooling occurs with the inability to swallow secretions. These children, who appear toxic at times, often sit quietly, leaning forward in an effort to create a sufficient airway.

Lateral films of the child's neck will show the typical edematous epiglottis and aryepiglottic folds; x-ray, however, is superfluous and may prove dangerous if the child is unnecessarily delayed in the radiology department. A recent prospective study has shown that epiglottitis can be differentiated from laryngotracheobronchitis by direct inspection of the epiglottis.[9] This study involved children in whom acute epiglottitis was suspected owing to the presence of drooling and the absence of a spontaneous cough. Examinations were performed only in the presence of an anesthesiologist who could intubate the patient. The authors felt that direct inspection of the epiglottis, initially with a tongue blade and then with a laryngoscope, could differentiate these conditions. They found no instances in 155 patients in which direct inspection precipitated

TABLE 4-1. Characteristics of Laryngotracheobronchitis and Epiglottitis

Characteristic	Laryngotracheobronchitis	Epiglottitis
Incidence	Common	Uncommon
Etiology	Viral	*Haemophilus influenzae* type B
Age	6 months to 3 years	2–6 years
Clinical picture	Gradual onset; preceding upper respiratory infection; barking cough	Rapid onset; fever; drooling; dysphagia
Physical examination	Respiratory distress, inspiratory stridor, low-grade temperature	Anxious; muffled voice, chin forward, drooling, high temperature
Laboratory	WBC usually <10,000/mm with lymphocytosis; x-ray shows narrowing of subglottic region	WBC often >10,000/mm with band cells increased; x-ray shows swollen epiglottis

Adapted from McLain LG: Croup syndrome. Am Fam Physician 36(4):213, 1987.

airway obstruction. All tests aside, however, the clinical picture of the child of age 2 or 3 years drooling, in respiratory distress, and feverish is sufficient to indicate epiglottitis.

Affected children should be taken to the operating room where an anesthesiologist can perform intubation; a surgeon skilled in endoscopy should be available in the event of a difficult intubation. The child is accompanied by a parent and given an inhalation anesthetic with high oxygen concentration. The larynx and supraglottic tissues are inspected and an orotracheal tube inserted. After cultures have been taken, the orotracheal tube is replaced by a soft polyvinyl tube, such as the opaque Portex tube, which is passed through the nose. The tube is uncuffed and one size smaller than usual. The epiglottis is usually very swollen and edematous, but the vocal cords and the larynx are seldom involved. The involvement of other supraglottic structures such as the false cords leads some to call this condition supraglottitis.[3] The infecting organism is usually *Haemophilus influenzae*. Intubation is commonly necessary only for 24 to 48 hours, and patients rapidly improve when the edema of the epiglottis subsides.[2,4] Neither racemic epinephrine nor steroids are helpful in the management of epiglottitis. Chloramphenicol and ampicillin are effective against *H. influenzae*, although a combination of sulbactam and ampicillin may prove safer.[5]

Table 4–1 lists the diagnostic as well as therapeutic features of spasmodic croup, laryngotracheobronchitis, bacterial tracheitis, and epiglottitis.[10] There remains, however, the need for some clarification in two controversial areas: the question of steroids and the argument surrounding tracheostomy versus intubation.

STEROIDS

The use of steroids in croup remains controversial.[1,7] Laboratory and clinical evidence has demonstrated the therapeutic efficacy of steroids in reducing edema in various inflammatory situations. Steroids are effective, however, *only when they are given early and in high doses.* In addition, steroids should be utilized only for a relatively short period of time, such as 48 to 72 hours. It is for these reasons that we use dexamethasone in high doses and for a limited period of time. The regimen probably helps; at the very least, it should do no harm if used for short periods. Dexamethasone, in a dose of 0.8 mg/kg/day (equivalent to 4 mg/kg/day of prednisone), is administered intravenously every 6 hours. Steroids are not given for epiglottitis and may prove harmful when used in conjunction with this condition.[8] The rationale for this therapeutic regimen with steroids is similar to that which we use in caustic inflammation of the esophagus.[12]

TRACHEOSTOMY VERSUS INTUBATION

Over the past 30 years, experience has shown that the trachea does not tolerate an endotracheal tube inserted through an inflamed glottis. With an inflammatory process involving the glottis, progressive edema may cause vascular compromise around an endotracheal tube and lead to necrosis in the subglottic area where the cartilaginous cricoid ring is unyielding. As swelling and inflammation progress, ulceration of the vocal cords and the subglottic area may develop. When faced with severe glottic inflammation, we prefer a temporary tracheostomy with extubation performed as the edema subsides.

Children with epiglottitis are another matter entirely. Inflammation of the glottic and subglottic regions does not occur with this condition, and intubation is well tolerated. Tracheostomy, therefore, is not required for patients with epiglottitis except in situations in which an endotracheal tube cannot be safely maintained for 24 hours, such as in hospitals in the tropics.[11] A review of patients at the Children's Hospital in Boston showed that endotracheal intubation by the nasotracheal route is safe and effective for the management of epiglottitis (or supraglottitis).[3] Others have noted the evolution from tracheostomy to endotracheal intubation.[14]

If a patient with relatively mild laryngotracheobronchitis (croup) without superimposed bacterial infection is intubated, no damage may result if the patient can be extubated within 48 hours. However, severe ulcerations of the larynx have occurred after only 24 hours of endotracheal intubation. The key to successful and safe endotracheal intubation is evaluation by the surgeon of the extent of inflammatory reaction in the glottic and subglottic regions. Endotracheal intubation may be well tolerated if edema is not extensive and if tubes of the proper size are used (Table 4–2).[13]

TABLE 4–2. Indications for Endotracheal Intubation and Tracheostomy

Clinical Situation	Endotracheal Intubation	Tracheostomy
Emergencies	Always, except →	Severe craniofacial or head and neck injuries
Neonates and infants <6 months	Oral intubation unless no hope of extubation →	When long-term intubation is required or when there is difficulty in maintaining intubation because of activity
Infants >6 months and children	Maintain for 7–14 days and then →	When long-term intubation or ventilatory support is required for conditions such as severe head injuries
Epiglottitis	Until infection has cleared	Usually not necessary
Croup or other severe glottic inflammatory diseases	If does not respond to inhalations of racemic epinephrine or with airway obstruction as a temporary measure before →	When glottic edema and inflammation are severe

REFERENCES

1. Asher MI, Beauedry PH: Croup and cortico-steroid therapy. J Pediatr 97:506–507, 1981
2. Butt W, Shann F, Walker C, et al.: Acute epiglottitis. A different approach to management. Crit Care Med 16:43–47, 1988
3. Crockett DM, McGill TJ, Healy GB, Friedman EM: Airway management of acute supraglottitis at the Children's Hospital, Boston: 1980–1985. Ann Otol Rhinol Laryngol 97:114–119, 1988
4. Gerber AC, Pfenninger J: Acute epiglottitis: Management by short duration of intubation and hospitalization. Intensive Care Med 12:407–411, 1986
5. Gonzalez C, Reilly JS, Kenna MA, Thompson AE: Duration of intubation in children with acute epiglottitis. Otolaryngol Head Neck Surg 95:477–481, 1986
6. Gussack GS, Tacchi EJ: Pulse oximetry in the management of pediatric airway disorders. South Med J 80:1381–1384, 1987
7. Hodge KM, Ganzel TM: Diagnostic and therapeutic efficiency in croup and epiglottitis. Laryngoscope 97:621–625, 1987
8. Kissoon N, Mitchell I: Adverse effects of racemic epinephrine in epiglottitis. Pediatr Emerg Care 1:143–144, 1985
9. Mauro RD, Poole SR, Lockhart CH: Differentiation of epiglottitis from laryngotracheitis in the child with stridor. Am J Dis Child 142:679–682, 1988
10. McLain LG: Croup syndrome. Am Fam Physician 36:207–214, 1987
11. Odetoyinbo O: A comparison of endotracheal intubation and tracheostomy in the management of acute epiglottitis in children in the tropics. J Laryngol Otol 100:1273–1278, 1986
12. Othersen HB Jr: Cardiothoracic injuries. In Touloukian RJ (ed): Pediatric Trauma. New York, John Wiley & Sons, 1978, pp 305–368
13. Othersen HB Jr: Intubation injuries of the trachea in children. Management and prevention. Ann Surg 189:601–606, 1979
14. Sendi K, Crysdale WS: Acute epiglottitis. A decade of change—a 10-year experience with 242 children. J Otolaryngol 16:196–202, 1987

part 2

Congenital and Acquired Problems

chapter 5

Subglottic Stenosis and Tracheobronchial Stricture: Classification and Therapy

H. Biemann Othersen, Jr., M.D.
C.D. Smith, M.D.

CLASSIFICATION

In any therapeutic endeavor it is important to have rules and definitions under which all participants operate. Thus, various treatments can be evaluated with a clear understanding that similar lesions are being compared. There is a need for such an approach in airway problems in children. Under the heading of "tracheal stenosis" or "subglottic stenosis," lesions are included that range from simple granulation and edema to the extreme of calcific scars or cartilaginous obstruction. To classify these diverse lesions, four different determinants of airway strictures must be included: location, etiology, type, and extent.

Location

Airway stenosis can be (Figure 5–1):
1. Laryngeal
   a. Supraglottic. Usually inflammatory diseases producing edema.
   b. Glottic. At the cords. Can be congenital or fibrotic after cord damage.
   c. Subglottic. Anywhere in the larynx from the true cords to the cricoid.
2. Subglottic. Usually located at the cricoid cartilage. This is the most common site for stenotic lesions in children since it is the narrowest point of the pediatric airway and the most unyielding lumen. As such it is the area in children most susceptible to damage.

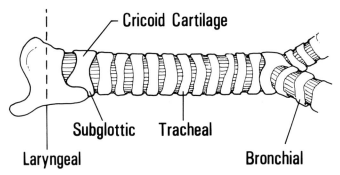

FIGURE 5-1. Sites of airway stenosis in children. The subglottic space at the cricoid is the narrowest point.

3. Tracheal. From the cricoid to the carina. Most lesions here in small children will be congenital, i.e., complete rings. In older children injury from an endotracheal cuff, a tracheostomy tube, or direct trauma is more common.
4. Bronchial. Airway distal to the carina. Usually inflammatory or induced by foreign bodies or neoplasms.

Etiology

1. Congenital. These strictures can occur in any of the locations described previously. There may be weblike strictures at the level of the cords and the larynx or blocks of cartilage completely obstructing the larynx. In the trachea, the subglottic area alone may be narrowed. In the remainder of the trachea complete cartilaginous rings without a membranous portion may produce long areas of stenosis.
2. Acquired. These stenotic lesions are usually the result of internal trauma produced by various endotracheal tubes. Usually a tube is too tight, and constriction at the cricoid results in a circumferential area of necrosis, which leads to ultimate scarring and stricture. Laryngotracheitis may produce edema and inflammation, making a normally fitting tube too tight. There also can be erosion at the site of impingement of the cuff on an endotracheal or tracheostomy tube. Finally, a tracheostomy tube produces erosion at the superior margin of the tracheal stoma and may ultimately lead to granulation and stenosis or to tracheomalacia.[6]

Type

There are five basic types of stenotic lesions:
1. Granulomatous. These lesions consist primarily of edematous granulation tissue. They represent the earliest of tracheal injuries and are the easiest to treat. (Fig. 5–2).
2. Fibrous. These stenotic lesions are usually smooth and rubbery and can be dilated but will return to their previous size after dilation has been completed. These well-established strictures are more difficult to treat (Fig. 5–3).

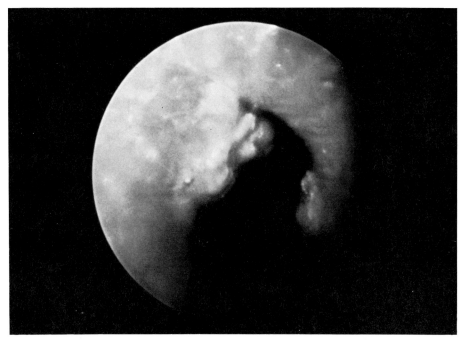

FIGURE 5–2. Bronchoscopic photograph of an acute airway injury showing the irregular granulation impingement.

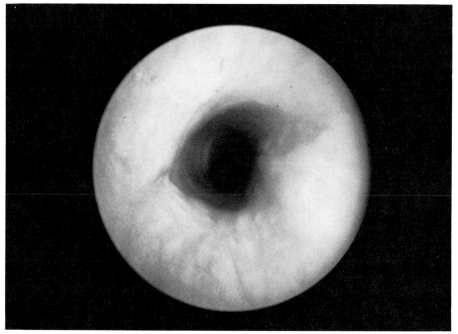

FIGURE 5–3. Bronchoscopic photograph of a chronic airway lesion showing the smooth fibrous narrowing.

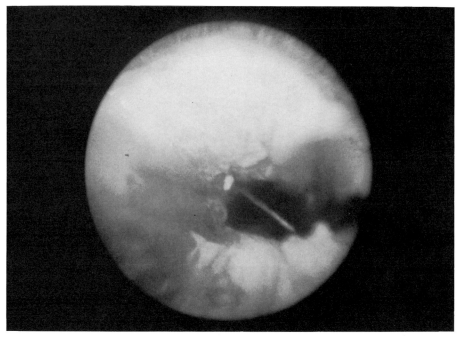

FIGURE 5-4. Bronchoscopic photograph of a chronic airway stenotic lesion that has progressed to calcification.

3. Calcific. These lesions appear irregular like the granulomatous lesions but are hard and firm and contain fibrous tissue as well as calcification, which makes them extremely rigid and difficult to dilate (Fig. 5–4).
4. Inflammatory. Any of the lesions described previously may be superimposed by inflammation complicating their treatment and resolution. The inflammation may be caused by an infection such as laryngotracheobronchitis; an irritation, such as inhalation of toxins or aspiration of gastric contents; or trauma, such as that induced by a foreign body or an endotracheal tube. It is usually impossible to relieve the stricture until the inflammation has been resolved (Fig. 5–5).
5. Cartilaginous. These lesions are congenital in nature and may consist of a complete block of cartilage that obstructs the laryngeal lumen, or more commonly, tracheal rings that are complete and without a membranous portion. This abnormality produces strictures of the trachea, which vary in extent and severity of the stenosis. These lesions usually require operative therapy, although there have been some reports of successful dilation (Fig. 5–6).

Extent

Flow of gases in the airway depends on the cross-sectional diameter of the tube (windpipe). An adequate description of a stenotic lesion must include the percentage reduction of the lumen. This figure should be expressed as a percentage of the cross-sectional area. To measure the airway diameter, a Fogarty catheter is inserted through the bronchoscope and inflated under direct vision. The catheter is placed in the normal part of the airway, and the amount of water

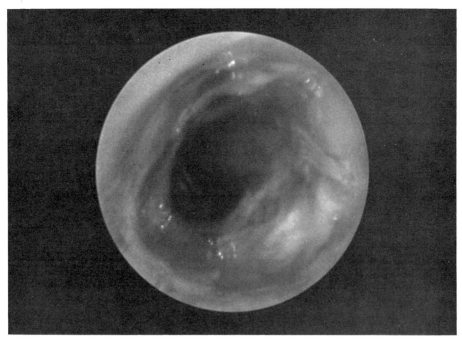

FIGURE 5–5. Bronchoscopic photograph of an inflamed airway. Stenotic lesions can have superimposed acute and chronic inflammation.

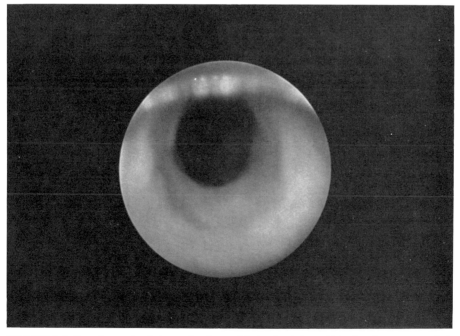

FIGURE 5–6. Bronchoscopic photograph of complete tracheal rings. Note the absence posteriorly of a membranous portion.

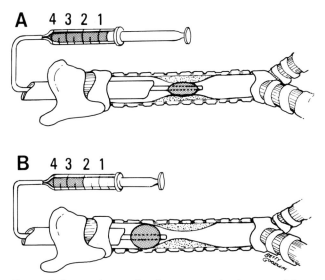

FIGURE 5-7. Fogarty balloon catheter inflated to measure the diameter of the airway stricture.

required to inflate the balloon to occlude the lumen is noted. The catheter is then positioned in the stenotic portion and the amount of water necessary to inflate the balloon to the diameter of the lumen is again determined (Fig. 5–7). The catheter is then removed and the balloon inflated with the previously determined amounts of water and the diameters of the inflated balloon measured. The diameters of the normal trachea and the stenotic segment can be determined. By dividing this figure in half the radius is obtained. Then using the formula; πr^2, the cross-sectional area can be determined for both segments.

In addition to the diameter of the stenosis, the length of the stricture must be determined. Again, a Fogarty catheter can be passed to the end of the stricture and the balloon inflated and pulled back against the stenotic segment. The length of the catheter at the bronchoscope is marked, the balloon deflated, and the catheter retracted to the proximal end of the stricture and again marked. The length of the stricture can then be determined (Fig. 5–8).

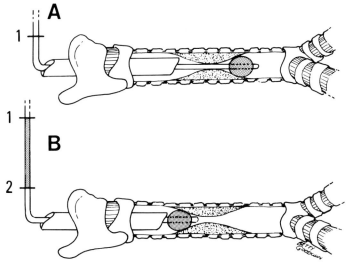

FIGURE 5-8. Use of Fogarty catheter to determine length of a stricture.

THERAPY

Therapy can be divided into adjunctive measures, endobronchial procedures (endoscopic tracheoplasty), and open operative laryngotracheoplasties.

1. Adjunctive measures include the following:
   a. Prevention of further inflammation or irritation by use of a smaller tube or by treatment of infection, etc.[3]
   b. Tracheostomy. This procedure may bypass the lesion, especially if the stenosis is in the subglottic area. A long tube can be utilized via the tracheostomy to pass through a stenotic lesion into the lower trachea. Tracheostomy is considered adjunctive since it does not improve the stenotic lesion itself.
   c. Steroid administration. Steroids can be given systemically or injected into the lesion itself. There is no good experimental or clinical evidence definitely proving the value of steroids when injected into a tracheal lesion. However, inference can be made from the use of intralesional injection of steroid into scars elsewhere in the body. Definite benefit has been shown with hypertrophic scars of the skin. The use of systemic steroids to reduce inflammatory processes is only slightly less controversial. For short-term use, there does seem to be a role for anti-inflammatory steroids.
2. Endoscopic maneuvers. Endoscopic tracheoplasty includes procedures that will benefit the stenotic lesion itself. Included are maneuvers such as balloon dilation[7] and endoscopic removal of obstructing lesions by laser, cryotherapy, or electrosurgical resection. Often these procedures are combined with steroids administered either systemically or injected intralesionally.[1,4,5] These endoscopic tracheoplasties are most efficacious in the granulomatous types of lesions where protruding granulation can be excised and the stenotic segment dilated with balloons. A short-term stent, consisting of a pliable endotracheal tube, can be inserted and utilized along with systemic steroids and antibiotics for 72 hours. At the end of that time extubation is accomplished with the help of racemic epinephrine inhalations and other measures to reduce edema. We have not had much success with balloon dilation of congenital tracheal rings or bronchial strictures.
3. Operative laryngotracheoplasties. These are direct operative procedures upon the trachea itself, including:
   a. A castellated incision with open excision of scar and insertion of an endotracheal stent, thus closing the trachea in an expanded position.[2]
   b. Tracheal resection and primary anastomosis. This procedure has not been utilized in children as often as in adults because of the fear of interference with tracheal growth. Recent studies have shown that, in children, much more of the trachea can be resected than was previously thought.
   c. Cartilage tracheoplasty. The stenotic segment is opened anteriorly and occasionally posteriorly with no attempt to resect the intraluminal scar. A portion of costal cartilage is inserted into the defect to expand the lumen. Other materials have been utilized to fill the gap. Portions of bone and periosteum and pericardium have all been attributed some success. All of these open tracheoplasties can be combined with various types of intraluminal stents, which have been utilized on a long- or short-term basis.

The various types of laryngoplasties and details of the procedures will be presented in subsequent chapters.

We do not include an enumeration of procedures and patients with airway problems. The guidelines presented here are based on extensive experience with over 100 children who have had congenital and acquired airway stenosis.

REFERENCES

1. Birk HG: Endoscopic repair of laryngeal stenosis. Trans Am Acad Ophthalmol Otol 74:140, 1970
2. Evans JNG: Laryngeal disorders in children. *In* Wilkinson AW (ed): Recent Advances in Pediatric Surgery. Edinburgh, Churchill Livingstone, 1975, p 174
3. Othersen HB Jr: Intubation injuries of the trachea in children—management and prevention. Ann Surg 189(5):601–606, 1979
4. Othersen HB Jr: Steroid therapy for tracheal stenosis in children. Ann Thorac Surg 17:254, 1974
5. Othersen HB Jr: The technique of intraluminal stenting and steroid administration in the treatment of tracheal stenosis in children. J Pediatr Surg 9:683, 1974
6. Othersen HB Jr: Trachea, lungs, and pleural cavity. *In* Welch KJ (ed): Complications in Pediatric Surgery: Prevention and Management. Philadelphia, W.B. Saunders Co., 1982, Chap 15
7. Othersen HB Jr, Leithiser RL, Powell DM, et al: Endoscopic tracheoplasty and esophagoplasty in children: A new technique utilizing balloon catheters. Unpublished data

chapter 6

Vascular Malformations with Airway Obstruction

Paul W. Braunstein, Jr., M.D.
Robert M. Sade, M.D.

Extrinsic compression of the airway by congenital anomalies of the major thoracic arteries is an important cause of airway obstruction in children. Although such malformations account for only 1% of all congenital cardiovascular anomalies, they may be the cause of 25% of the airway obstructions seen by pediatric thoracic surgeons.[11] In this chapter we review the anatomy, clinical features, diagnosis, and surgical treatment of the constellation of vascular anomalies causing airway obstruction.

EMBRYOGENESIS

The thoracic great arteries normally develop from the primitive ventral and dorsal aortas, which are connected by six pairs of aortic arches. Arch pairs 1, 2, and 5 disappear, whereas arch pair 3 becomes the common and internal carotid arteries. The right 4th arch becomes the innominate artery, and the left 4th arch becomes the aortic arch. Arch pair 6 forms the proximal branch pulmonary arteries and ducti arteriosi.[33]

In 1953, Edwards diagrammed the concept of a stage of aortic development at which there is a double aortic arch with bilateral ducti (Fig. 6–1A).[26] The normal aorta and all the arch anomalies can be easily derived from this conceptual diagram. Resorption of specific portions of the arches may account for most of the congenital aortic arch anomalies (Fig. 6–1B through G).

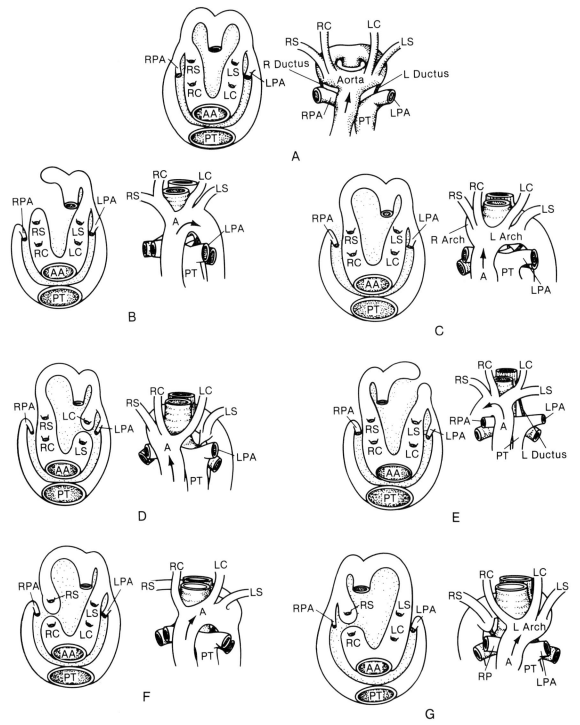

FIGURE 6-1. Aortic arch anomalies. *A,* Conceptualized pattern of primitive aortic arches and branches. Development of (*B*) normal left arch, (*C*) double arch, (*D*) right arch with aberrant left subclavian artery, (*E*) right arch with mirror image branching and left ductus arteriosus, (*F*) left arch with aberrant right subclavian artery with left ductus arteriosus, and (*G*) left arch with aberrant right subclavian artery with right ductus arteriosus (mirror image of *D*). *A,* aorta; *AA,* ascending aorta; *AS,* aortic sac; *LC,* left common carotid artery; *L Ductus,* left ductus arteriosus; *LPA,* left pulmonary artery; *LS,* left subclavian artery; *LV,* left ventricle; *L Arch,* left aortic arch; *PT,* pulmonary arterial trunk; *RC,* right common carotid artery; *R Ductus,* right ductus arteriosus; *RPA,* right pulmonary artery; *RS,* right subclavian artery; *RV,* right ventricle; *R Arch,* right aortic arch.

GENERAL APPROACH TO DIAGNOSIS

In a child with a suspected vascular ring, the presence and anatomy of the ring can be suggested by the anteroposterior (AP) and lateral x-rays of the chest. Findings may include shadows typical of a right or left aortic arch, deviation of the trachea to the left produced by a right aortic arch or to the right by a left arch, and anterior tracheal compression.

The barium esophagogram is an important diagnostic tool. It may demonstrate extrinsic compression that can be diagnostic for several types of vascular rings. Plain chest x-ray and barium esophagogram may establish the definitive diagnosis in around 90% of patients. Because nearly all vascular rings can be surgically approached by way of a left thoracotomy and dissection of the vessels will clearly expose the anatomy, some surgeons believe these simple studies alone are necessary preoperatively.

Aortography, however, may provide a more precise definition of the anatomy, including stenotic and atretic zones, so it is often used during preoperative evaluation. In addition, McFaul and colleagues felt that preoperative aortography avoided a "wrong-sided" left thoracotomy in 10 to 20% of their patients with vascular rings.[20] Aortography may be helpful in evaluating the 12 to 15% incidence of congenital heart disease in infants with vascular rings, although in recent years echocardiography has become increasingly definitive in the elucidation of intracardiac malformations. Aortography is generally quite safe, but there is a finite, although small, morbidity in the pediatric age group; digital subtraction angiography has therefore been recommended as a less invasive alternative to catheterization that yields equivalent information.[23,35]

Noninvasive evaluation of congenital abnormalities of the thoracic aorta has been greatly enhanced by the use of computed tomography (CT),[22] two-dimensional echocardiography,[36] and magnetic resonance imaging (MRI).[6] CT with contrast has been shown to be accurate in the diagnosis of vascular rings and slings but requires a large amount of radiation to obtain precise information. Two-dimensional echocardiography and color flow Doppler have been refined in recent years and have become valuable diagnostic adjuncts. They avoid the morbidity of aortography and digital subtraction angiography and the radiation of CT. Echocardiography has been shown to be fairly accurate in diagnosing vascular rings and other congenital heart abnormalities. MRI may accurately show the malformation in children with vascular rings, but the technique is limited to two-dimensional transverse plane slices of the thorax, so it may not produce clear visual definition of the three-dimensional anomaly. It may become more useful when three-dimensional image reconstruction becomes generally available. Echocardiography and MRI may eventually become the procedures of choice in the diagnosis of vascular rings.[32]

The role of bronchoscopy is not generally established. It may be helpful in children with suspected tracheomalacia and is clearly useful in those with anomalous innominate artery[11] and pulmonary artery sling.[29] Bronchoscopy may localize the site of compression and the severity of tracheomalacia and may be used postoperatively to assure that correction of the airway compression is achieved. Patients with pulmonary artery sling have a high incidence (50%) of severe tracheobronchial abnormalities that may be delineated with bronchoscopy.

Contrast tracheobronchography has been advocated as the primary diagnostic tool in evaluating airway obstruction, but it may be associated with acute airway edema and obstruction, particularly if water-soluble contrast material

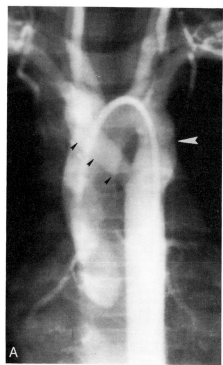
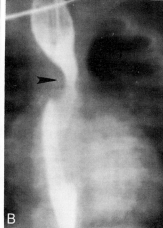
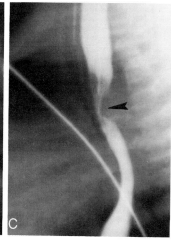

FIGURE 6-2. Double aortic arch. *A,* Arch aortogram in the AP projection demonstrates the anterior (left) arch (white arrowhead) and posterior (right) arch (black arrowheads). *B,* Barium esophagogram demonstrates the right posterior esophageal compression by the right aortic arch (arrowhead) in the AP projection. *C,* Same as *B,* but lateral projection.

enters the alveoli.[9] We have therefore limited its use to situations in which anatomic malformations are suspected and cannot be clearly defined by bronchoscopy alone: for example, in determining the distal extent of tracheobronchial hypoplasia associated with complete tracheal rings in pulmonary artery sling.[31]

AORTIC ARCH MALFORMATIONS

Double Aortic Arch

In 1937, Hommel was the first to describe a double aortic arch. In 1945, Gross was the first to perform successful surgery. It is by far the most common (40%) of the aortic rings.

ANATOMY

The ascending aorta arises normally and bifurcates into two arches (Fig. 6–2*A;* see also Fig. 6–1*C*). The anterior branch (left aortic arch) proceeds leftward over the anterior wall of the trachea and posteriorly over the left main bronchus, and receives the ligamentum or ductus arteriosus, before joining the descending aorta. The posterior branch (right aortic arch) curves posteriorly over the right main bronchus, proceeds behind the esophagus, and joins the left anterior arch to complete the formation of the descending aorta. The origin of each carotid and subclavian artery is on the corresponding arch. The important variables of the anatomy are the relative size of the lumen of each arch, the patency of each arch, and the sidedness of the upper descending aorta and the ductus arteriosus. In 70 to 90% of cases, the right arch is dominant and the left arch may be hypoplastic or atretic anywhere along its course. When the left arch is dominant, the right can be hypoplastic or atretic at any point. A double aortic arch usually exists as an isolated anomaly, although associated congenital heart disease has been reported.[21]

CLINICAL FEATURES

Almost all infants with double aortic arch are symptomatic, and the severity of symptoms depends upon the tightness of the vascular ring encircling the trachea and esophagus. Symptoms are usually present at birth or soon thereafter and can include coughing, mild stridor with wheezing, and attacks of dyspnea and cyanosis. Reflex apnea may occur; this is characterized by reflex respiratory arrest initiated by either a bolus of food passing through the esophagus or accumulation of tracheobronchial secretions. These children may present with feeding difficulties, recurrent respiratory infections, or a history of holding the neck extended (flexion usually increases respiratory distress; extension decreases it).

DIAGNOSIS

Definition of the anomaly as a double aortic arch is difficult on chest roentgenogram, which may demonstrate the dominant arch. The lateral chest x-ray may disclose narrowing of the trachea at or above the carina. Barium esophagogram usually shows two esophageal indentations at two different levels and of unequal caliber (Fig. 6–2B and C), the larger indentation being produced by the dominant arch, usually the right. Nuclear MRI, arch aortography, digital subtraction angiography, and echocardiography have all been utilized in confirming the diagnosis and planning surgical therapy.

SURGICAL THERAPY

The indication for operative correction is severity of symptoms. Patients with few or no symptoms do not require surgery, because it is unlikely that symptoms will develop as the patient ages. Most patients are symptomatic enough to require surgery, however, and the anomaly is approached through a 4th left intercostal space posterolateral thoracotomy. Phrenic, vagus, and recurrent laryngeal nerves should be preserved. The ring must be completely dissected free from mediastinal structures and the hypoplastic arch identified. When the anterior left arch is hypoplastic, it should be divided at its most hypoplastic segment. When the posterior right arch is hypoplastic, it should be divided at its most hypoplastic segment, usually behind the esophagus, just proximal to its junction with the descending aorta. The ligamentum or ductus must be divided.[2] To ensure that the fibrous tissues surrounding the esophagus and trachea are not contributing to the compromise of the airway, all fibrous tissue on the surface of the esophagus should be divided. If tracheomalacia is identified by bronchoscopy or inspection at surgery, the ascending aorta can be sewn to the sternum or anterior chest wall, serving to decompress the trachea and pull it into an open position.

Right Aortic Arch with Mirror Image Branching and Left Ductus Arteriosus

ANATOMY

The ascending aorta passes upward and to the right anterior to the trachea, then curves over the right main bronchus and descends posteriorly (see Fig. 6–1E). The branches from the aortic arch are the mirror image of the normal left aortic arch: the first branch is the left innominate artery, followed by the right carotid and the right subclavian. The ductus in this anomaly is usually left-sided but may be right-sided or bilateral. When on the left, the ductus may connect the left pulmonary artery to the left subclavian artery, leaving the vascular ring incomplete, or it can connect the left pulmonary artery to the descending aorta and pull the aorta anteriorly against the trachea and esophagus.[27] Congenital intracardiac anomalies are often associated with the right aortic arch and almost always (98%) when there is mirror image branching. Right aortic arch may be associated with tetralogy of Fallot in 30% of those cases, double outlet right ventricle (20%), or truncus arteriosus (30%), among others.[21]

CLINICAL FEATURES

If a left-sided ductus is present between the left pulmonary artery and left subclavian artery, the vascular ring is open, so symptoms of vascular compression are not common, and other symptoms are usually due to the associated congenital heart disease. If the left ductus attaches the left pulmonary artery to the descending aorta, symptoms similar to those of the double aortic arch may be present but usually are not as severe and have later onset.

DIAGNOSIS

The chest x-ray typically shows a right aortic arch with no vascular shadow where the left aortic knob usually is seen. The esophagogram usually shows an indentation on the right side of the esophagus; a posterior esophageal compression may be present when the left ductus lies between the left pulmonary artery and descending aorta.

SURGICAL THERAPY

Through a left posterolateral thoracotomy, the ligamentum or ductus is interrupted and any fibrous tissue on the trachea and the esophagus is divided.

Right Aortic Arch with Aberrant Left Subclavian Artery

ANATOMY

This anomaly results from regression of the left 4th arch between the left carotid and left subclavian (see Fig. 6–1D). The first branch of the ascending aorta is the left carotid artery, followed by the right carotid and right subclavian arteries. The left subclavian artery arises as the last branch, and its point of origin is often bulbous (Kommerele's diverticulum). The retroesophageal component of the vascular ring can be the aorta when it descends to the left of the spine or the left subclavian artery when the arch descends to the right. The ductus arteriosus or ligamentum completes the ring; it is usually left sided and connects the left subclavian artery to the left pulmonary artery. Congenital heart defects are unusual with this anomaly.

CLINICAL FEATURES

Symptoms are quite variable. Respiratory symptoms are more common than esophageal. Cough, noisy breathing, dyspnea, and stridor are the most common symptoms. Most infants present shortly after birth, and symptoms are often much milder than those of infants with double aortic arch. Surgery is required in only 10 to 30% of children with this anomaly.[10]

DIAGNOSIS

The chest x-ray usually reveals a normal cardiac configuration with the shadow of a right-sided arch. The AP esophagogram usually demonstrates a small left indentation (subclavian artery) and a small right indentation (aortic arch). The lateral esophagogram, however, may show a large posterior indentation owing to the bulbous origin of the subclavian artery (Kommerele's diverticulum) (Fig. 6–3).

SURGICAL TREATMENT

Through a left posterolateral thoracotomy, the pleura lateral to the esophagus and left subclavian artery is opened. The ligamentum arteriosum and the left subclavian artery are completely mobilized. The ligamentum or the ductus is divided. The contribution of the aberrant left subclavian artery to the symptoms

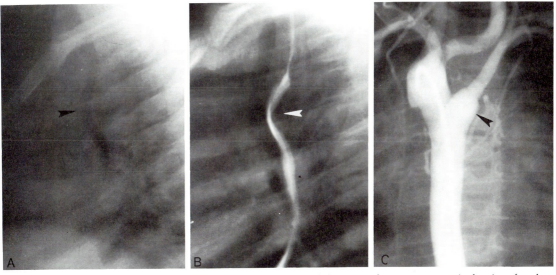

FIGURE 6–3. Right arch and aberrant left subclavian artery. *A,* Lateral chest x-ray demonstrates anterior bowing of trachea (arrowhead). *B,* Lateral projection of barium-lined esophagus shows posterior indentation due to the bulbous origin of the subclavian artery (Kommerele's diverticulum). *C,* Aortic arch angiogram demonstrates the aberrant left subclavian and Kommerele's diverticulum (arrowhead) in the AP projection.

of the ring is often uncertain, but to avoid residual symptoms we divide the left subclavian artery at its origin. Although some advocate reanastomosis of the subclavian, we believe this unnecessarily complicates the procedure since interruption of the subclavian artery is well tolerated. We have never observed postoperative subclavian steal syndrome, but should this occur late after the operation, the subclavian can be revascularized at that time.[24]

Others believe the left subclavian artery should be divided and, in older children and adults, reanastomosed to the aorta or the left common carotid.

Aberrant Right Subclavian Artery with Left Ductus Arteriosus

ANATOMY

In this anomaly, the right subclavian arises as the last branch of the aortic arch and courses from left to right to reach the right arm (see Fig. 6–1F). The artery courses from left to right posterior to the esophagus but has been reported rarely to pass between the esophagus and trachea or anterior to the trachea. The ligamentum or ductus is usually left sided. The aberrant vessel does not form a complete ring but indents the posterior esophagus. There appears to be a higher incidence of this lesion in patients with coarctation of the aorta and in those with Down's syndrome associated with congenital heart disease.[13]

Rarely, the ligamentum or ductus is right sided, in which case it is the mirror image (and clinically behaves the same) of right aortic arch with aberrant left subclavian artery (see previous discussion and Fig. 6–1G).

CLINICAL PRESENTATION

Respiratory symptoms are rarely present during childhood, but dysphagia may appear later in life. Most often, though, patients with this lesion remain asymptomatic throughout life.

DIAGNOSIS

The chest x-ray is normal, without evidence of tracheal compression. The esophagogram demonstrates findings that are virtually diagnostic of this syndrome. In the AP projection, the artery produces an oblique linear defect in the esophagus. The lateral projection demonstrates a wedge-shaped defect seen on the posterior esophageal wall at or below the level of the aortic arch. Since this lesion is rarely symptomatic, the presence of dysphagia demands investigation of intrinsic esophageal disease.

SURGICAL TREATMENT

Operation may be needed in the rare patient who is severely symptomatic. In infants the approach is through a left thoracotomy and the ligamentum and right subclavian artery are divided at their origins. In older children and adults, a right thoracotomy may be used. After division of the aberrant right subclavian artery, it may be anastomosed to the right carotid artery or aortic arch.[18] Alternatively, the vertebral artery may be ligated to prevent subclavian steal. In the rare case of right-sided ligamentum or ductus, the approach is through a right thoracotomy. The ligamentum or ductus is interrupted, and any fibrous tissue on the trachea and esophagus is divided.

Left Aortic Arch with Aberrant Innominate Artery

ANATOMY

This is not a vascular ring, but the innominate artery arises further leftward (Fig. 6–4A), and therefore more posteriorly than normal, and compresses the trachea anteriorly (Fig. 6–4B). In fact, it has been observed that the innominate artery need not be aberrant or anomalous to compress the trachea. Infants who have had repair of esophageal atresia or tracheoesophageal fistula are at particular risk of severe anterior tracheal compression by the innominate artery. The trachea is abutted posteriorly by the dysmotile esophagus and thereby displaced anteriorly against the innominate artery. Tracheomalacia is a common consequence of the anterior compression.

Anomalous left carotid artery is a very rare anomaly, but its presentation, diagnosis, and treatment are the same as those of the anomalous left innominate artery.[15]

CLINICAL PRESENTATION

Those who are symptomatic may present with episodes of reflex apnea or recurrent respiratory infection.[3] Cough, stridor, pneumonia, and, less commonly,

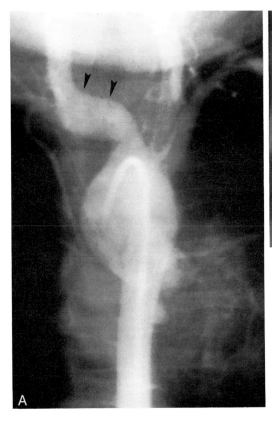

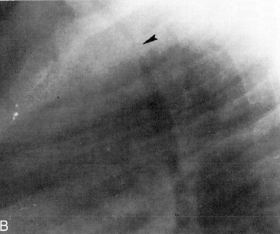

FIGURE 6–4. Aberrant innominate artery. *A,* Angiographic demonstration of the aberrant innominate artery (arrowheads) overlying the air-filled trachea. *B,* Lateral chest x-ray reveals tracheal compression by the innominate artery (arrowhead).

wheezing, cyanosis, and noisy breathing may also be seen. The average age at onset of symptoms is approximately 9 months.

DIAGNOSIS

The lateral chest x-ray may demonstrate anterior tracheal compression (Fig. 6–4B). Barium esophagogram is normal. When this anomaly is suspected, bronchoscopy is useful to visualize tracheal compression that pulsates and courses upward from left to right anteriorly, about 1 to 2 cm above the carina. Anterior displacement of the bronchoscope usually obliterates the right radial and temporal pulses. Tracheomalacia usually occurs beneath the compressing artery and may be seen during bronchoscopy.

A noninvasive method that may document the degree of tracheal compression is measurement of flow-volume loop patterns, which are specific and reproducible for intra- and extrathoracic airway obstruction.[1,19]

SURGICAL TREATMENT

Anterior tracheal indentation may be seen in as many as 30% of randomly selected lateral chest x-rays of normal children,[34] so the mere association of this finding with respiratory symptoms is not sufficient to justify operation. For children who have few or no symptoms (approximately 80 to 90%), conservative medical therapy, including humidified oxygen and appropriate antibiotics when indicated, may be sufficient. This therapy will usually lead to gradual improvement of symptoms over a period of months to years as tracheal rigidity increases.

Surgical correction should be elected for patients with severe symptoms, reflex apnea, recurrent severe respiratory infection, or high-grade obstruction (more than 50% tracheal narrowing at bronchoscopy). Infants with previous esophageal atresia or tracheoesophageal fistula repair are at high risk for life-threatening reflex apnea and respond very well to surgery, so indications for operation in these infants should be less stringent.[30]

The surgical treatment of choice is innominate or ascending aortic arteriopexy to the sternum or anterior chest wall.[8] A left or right anterior thoracotomy through the 3rd or 4th intercostal space is utilized. The dissection ideally should be extrapleural and the ipsilateral thymic lobe should be excised, taking great care to preserve the phrenic nerve. The tissue plane between the aortic arch and trachea is not dissected since this attachment may stent the anterior wall of the trachea when the vessel is suspended. Nonabsorbable sutures supported by pledgets should be utilized. Relief of compression after arteriopexy can be confirmed by intraoperative bronchoscopy.

Results are excellent for patients with reflex apnea, particularly after previous tracheoesophageal fistula repair. Patients with less severe symptoms are not as likely to benefit from the procedure.

Rare Aortic Arch Anomalies

An aberrant left innominate artery arising as the 3rd branch of the right aortic arch and passing retroesophageal has been reported.[14] Origin of the left subclavian artery from the ductus or an atretic portion of aorta (leading to isolation of the left subclavian from the aortic blood flow) is also an uncommon anomaly.[4]

A vascular ring formed by the right pulmonary artery of a hemitruncal pulmonary artery as it courses to the right between the trachea and esophagus has been described. Binet and coworkers described an anomalous vessel from the right pulmonary artery origin crossing to the left between the esophagus and trachea to enter the descending aorta adjacent to the origin of an anomalous right subclavian artery. They named this a ductus arteriosus sling.[5]

PULMONARY ARTERY SLING

Since the original description by Glaevecke and Doehle in 1897,[12] the aberrant left pulmonary artery has become recognized as a distinct entity among the vascular anomalies causing airway obstruction.

Embryogenesis (Fig. 6–5)[22]

The lung bud appears in the 3-mm embryo as a ventral outpouching of the primitive foregut. As the bud develops, it carries with it a blood supply derived from the splanchnic plexus, the "pulmonary postbranchial plexus." The 6th aortic arches are formed by the conjunction of ventral buds from the aortic sac and dorsal buds from the dorsal aorta. As the ventral and dorsal buds grow toward each other, a branch is sent from each ventral bud to the pulmonary postbranchial plexus, completing the primitive main branch pulmonary arteries.

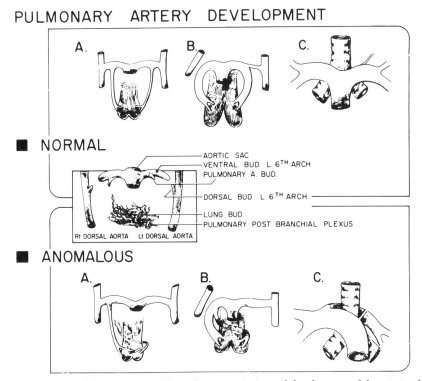

FIGURE 6–5. Normal development of the pulmonary arteries and development of the retrotracheal anomalous left pulmonary artery (see text for explanation).

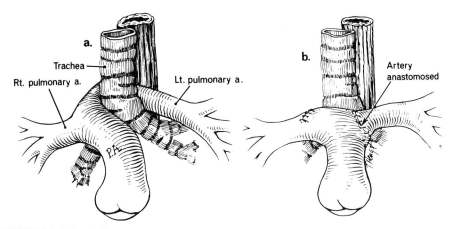

FIGURE 6-6. Surgical correction of pulmonary artery sling. *A,* Anatomy of the malformation. *B,* Surgical repair. Division and reanastomosis of the anomalous vessel to the main pulmonary artery. (Reprinted with permission from Cooley D, Wukasch D: Techniques in Vascular Surgery. Philadelphia, W.B. Saunders Co., 1979.)

On the right side the dorsal contribution to the 6th arch completely disappears, but on the left it persists as the ductus arteriosus.

If the left pulmonary plexus fails to connect with the left 6th arch, it may capture its arterial supply by connection through the postbranchial plexus with the derivatives of the right 6th aortic arch. This connection can be established through capillaries cephalad or caudad to the lung bud. If the cephalic connection is established, the connection is in front of the developing lung bud and the anatomic result is indistinguishable from normal anatomy except that the ductus arteriosus does not arise from the origin of the left pulmonary artery but from the main pulmonary artery proximal to the origin of the left pulmonary artery. If, however, the caudad plexus establishes connection with the right pulmonary artery as the lung bud develops, the course of the left pulmonary artery is behind the developing tracheobronchial tree, resulting in pulmonary artery sling.

Anatomy

A pulmonary artery sling occurs when the left pulmonary artery arises from the right pulmonary artery (Fig. 6–6*A*). The anomalous vessel passes posteriorly over the right main bronchus near its origin, turns to the left, crosses the mediastinum between the trachea and esophagus, and enters the hilum of the left lung. This produces a sling around the right mainstem bronchus and lower trachea, often compressing these structures. Congenital anomalies are associated in one half to two thirds of the cases and primarily involve the tracheobronchial tree or cardiovascular system.[29]

The most important associated tracheobronchial abnormality is hypoplasia of the distal trachea or mainstem bronchus or some combination of these. The tracheal stenosis is often associated with complete cartilaginous rings. Bronchus suis (right upper lobe or segmental bronchus arising directly from the trachea) may also be seen.

Congenital cardiovascular anomalies are associated with pulmonary artery sling in one half the cases and may include atrial septal defect, patent ductus arteriosus, tetralogy of Fallot, aortic stenosis, left superior vena cava, and aortic arch anomalies. Other associated anomalies have been described involving the gastrointestinal, genitourinary, and endocrine systems.

Clinical Presentation

The most common symptoms are those of respiratory obstruction, characterized by stridor and wheezing. The obstruction is greatest during expiration, in contrast to patients with aortic arch anomalies, whose obstruction is inspiratory and often involves the esophagus. Most patients, approximately 80%, will be symptomatic and about two thirds will present within the first few months or first year of life.

Diagnosis

The plain chest x-ray may demonstrate unequal aeration due to bronchial compression or stenosis, a low left hilum because the left pulmonary artery is behind and under rather than above the left bronchus, anterior bowing of the right main bronchus as it is pushed forward by the anomalous vessel behind it, deviation of the lower trachea and carina to the left (Fig. 6–7A), diminished size of the left pulmonary artery branches, and a mediastinal mass between the trachea and esophagus. Barium esophagogram characteristically shows an anterior indentation located at the lower trachea or carina that has an oblique angulation toward the right shoulder (Fig. 6–7B). Occasionally, the esophagus will be completely normal.

Since there is a high incidence of associated tracheobronchial abnormalities, preoperative assessment of the tracheobronchial tree is necessary and can be performed by endoscopy, airway fluoroscopy, contrast tracheography, or a

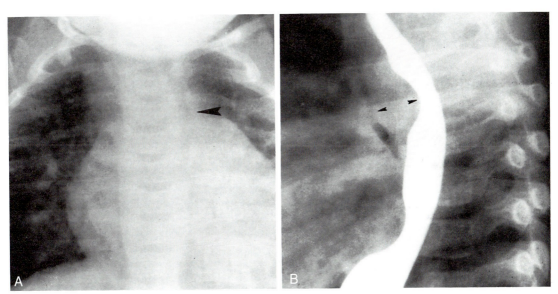

FIGURE 6–7. Pulmonary artery sling. *A,* Plain AP chest x-ray showing the lower trachea and carina being pulled to the left by the anomalous right pulmonary artery (arrowhead). *B,* Lateral projection of a barium esophagogram showing anterior displacement of the trachea and posterior compression of the esophagus by the anomalous vessel (arrowheads).

combination of these. It is extremely important to assess the severity and degree of associated tracheobronchial abnormalities because postoperative mortality is highly correlated with associated lesions. Two-dimensional echocardiography[32] and CT[25] have been utilized to confirm the diagnosis. Although the diagnosis can be established by noninvasive means, arteriography may be useful in confirming the anatomy as well as evaluating associated congenital heart abnormalities. Injection should be into the main pulmonary artery rather than a more proximal site because the anomalous vessel can be missed with proximal injection.

Surgical Treatment

Conservative medical treatment results in a mortality rate of 90%. Operation is indicated in all cases.[29]

The surgical approach may be through a median sternotomy or left posterolateral thoracotomy. Median sternotomy has been advocated because it can be carried out easily, ventilatory compromise is avoided, and tracheal resection can be performed, if necessary.[7,16,17] This approach should be used if simultaneous correction of cardiac anomalies with cardiopulmonary bypass is planned.

Left thoracotomy is most often used, however, because it is easy to mobilize the trachea, esophagus, pulmonary hilum, and left pulmonary artery through this approach. After division of the ligamentum arteriosum, the left pulmonary artery can be dissected behind the trachea, divided near its take-off from the right pulmonary artery, and reimplanted into the main pulmonary artery (see Fig. 6–6B). The length of left pulmonary artery to be implanted into the main pulmonary artery should be carefully calibrated to prevent kinking by too long a vessel, which has been described as an operative complication. In the past, postoperative thrombosis or stenosis of the reconstructed left pulmonary artery occurred in about one half the patients, but with improved microsurgical techniques and selective use of systemic heparinization, this patency rate has markedly improved.

Because much of the postoperative morbidity and mortality is due to associated tracheobronchial lesions, concomitant tracheal resection for severe stenosis or aortopexy should be carried out if there is evidence of important tracheomalacia.[16] The use of cardiopulmonary bypass has been recommended to facilitate repair of combined lesions. Alternatively, such patients may undergo correction of the sling only, be treated with postoperative ventilatory support, and, if prolonged owing to respiratory insufficiency, undergo a second operation to correct the tracheobronchial lesion.

POSTOPERATIVE MANAGEMENT

Postoperative care of patients who have had airway obstruction requires meticulous attention to the respiratory tract. Patients who have good relief of their airway compression can usually be extubated soon after operation and require routine pulmonary toilet and humidified oxygen for several days.[28]

An occasional patient, however, will require prolonged ventilatory support. Ventilator dependency may be due to an associated anatomic tracheobronchial lesion, such as tracheobronchial hypoplasia and complete tracheal rings often seen in pulmonary artery sling or, more commonly, tracheomalacia produced by long standing tracheal compression by the vascular anomaly. A serious tracheobronchial lesion may not become clinically evident until the need for prolonged ventilatory support is manifested. Bronchoscopy and airway fluoroscopy are usually sufficient to define the nature of the residual airway disease, if it is not already known.

If copious secretions prevent early extubation, nutrition is an important part of long-term ventilatory support. Tube feedings, either gastric or duodenal, are begun 2 days after surgery (or hyperalimentation if the gut is not ready for feeding), and advanced to full nutritional support within 1 to 2 days.

Weaning from the ventilator and extubation follow routine protocol. If extubation is not possible, surgical interventions may include direct attack on anatomically correctable lesions or tracheostomy.

REFERENCES

1. Abramson AL, Goldstein MN, Stenzler A, Steele A: The use of tidal breathing flow volume loop in laryngotracheal disease of neonates and infants. Laryngoscope 92:922–926, 1982
2. Arciniegas E, Hakimi M, Hertzler JH, Farooki ZQ, Green EW: Surgical management of congenital vascular rings. J Thorac Cardiovasc Surg 77:721–727, 1979
3. Ardito JM, Tucker GF, Ossoff RH, DeLeon SY: Innominate artery compression of the trachea in infants with reflex apnea. Ann Otol 89:401–405, 1980
4. Ben-Shachar G, Bedor SD, Liebman J, Van Heeckeren D: Hemitruncal sling: A newly recognized anomaly and its surgical correction. J Thorac Cardiovasc Surg 90:146–148, 1985
5. Binet JP, Conso JF, Losay J: Ductus arteriosus sling: report of a newly recognized anomaly and its surgical correction. Thorax 33:72–75, 1978
6. Bisset GS, Strife JL, Kirks DR, Bailey WW: Vascular rings: Magnetic resonance imaging. AJR 149:251–256, 1987
7. Campbell DN, Lilly JR, Heiser JC, Clarke SR: The surgery of pulmonary artery "sling." J Pediatr Surg 18:855–856, 1983
8. Clevenger FW, Othersen HB, Smith CD: Relief of tracheal compression by aortopexy. Ann Thorac Surg, in press
9. Corno A, Giamberti A, Giannico S, et al: Airway obstructions associated with congenital heart disease in infancy. J Thorac Cardiovasc Surg, 99:1091–1098, 1990
10. Felson B, Palayew MJ: The two types of right aortic arch. Radiology 81:745–759, 1963
11. Filston HC, Ferguson TB Jr, Ordham HN: Airway obstruction by vascular anomalies. Importance of telescopic bronchoscopy. Ann Surg 205:541–549, 1987
12. Glaevecke, Doehle: Uber eine seltene eingeboborene Anomalie der Pulmonalarterie. Munch Med Wochnschr 44:950, 1897
13. Goldskin WB: Aberrant right subclavian in mongolism. AJR 95:131–134, 1965
14. Grollman JH, Bedynek JL, Henderson HS, Hall RJ: Right aortic arch with an aberrant retroesophageal innominate artery: Angiographic diagnosis. Radiology 90:782–783, 1968
15. Gross RE, Neuhauser E: Compression of the trachea and esophagus by vascular anomalies. Pediatrics 7:69–88, 1951
16. Hickey MStJ, Woods AE: Pulmonary artery sling with tracheal stenosis: One stage repair. Ann Thorac Surg 44:416–419, 1987
17. Jonas RA, Spevak PJ, McGill T, Castaneda AR: Pulmonary artery sling: Primary repair by tracheal resection in infancy. J Thorac Cardiovasc Surg 97:548–550, 1989
18. Kalke BR, Magotra R, Doshi SM: A new surgical approach to the management of symptomatic aberrant right subclavian artery. Ann Thorac Surg 44:86–89, 1987
19. Marmon LM, Bye MR, Haas JM, Balsara RK, Dunn JM: Vascular rings and slings: Long-term follow-up of pulmonary function. J Pediatr Surg 19:683–692, 1984
20. McFaul R, Millard P, Nowicki E: Vascular rings necessitating right thoracotomy. J Thorac Cardiovasc Surg 82:306–309, 1981
21. Moes CF: Vascular rings and anomalies of the aortic arch. *In* Keith J, Rowe R, Vlad P (eds): Heart Disease in Infancy and Childhood. New York, MacMillan Publishing Co., 1979, pp 856–881
22. Moncada R, Demos TC, Churchill R, Reynes C: Chronic stridor in a child: CT diagnosis of pulmonary vascular sling. J Comput Assist Tomogr 7:713–715, 1983
23. Otero-Cagide M, Moodie DS, Sterba R, Gill CC: Digital subtraction angiography in the diagnosis of vascular rings. Am Heart J 112:1304–1308, 1986
24. Pass HI, Sade RM: Tracheo-esophageal compressive syndromes of vascular origin. In Glenn WW (ed): Thoracic and Cardiovascular Surgery, 4th ed. New York, Appleton-Century-Crofts, 1982, pp 669–710

25. Rheuban KS, Ayers N, Still JG, Alford B: Pulmonary artery sling: A new diagnostic tool and clinical review. Pediatrics 69:472–475, 1982
26. Richardson JV, Doty DB, Rossi NP, Ehrenhaft JL: Operation for aortic arch anomalies. Ann Thorac Surg 31:426–432, 1981
27. Roesler M, de Leval M, Chrispin A, Stark J: Surgical management of vascular ring. Ann Surg 197:139–146, 1983
28. Sade RM, Cosgrove D, Casteneda A: Infant and Child Care in Heart Surgery. Chicago, Year Book Medical Publishers, 1977
29. Sade RM, Rosenthal A, Fellows K, Casteneda A: Pulmonary artery sling. J Thorac Cardiovasc Surg 69:333–346, 1975
30. Schwartz Z, Filler RM: Tracheal compression as a cause of apnea following repair of tracheo-esophageal fistula: Treatment by aortopexy. J Pediatr Surg 15:842–848, 1980
31. Siegel MJ, Shackelford GD, McAlister WH: Tracheobronchography in the evaluation of anomalous left pulmonary artery. Pediatr Radiol 12:235–238, 1982
32. Soulen RL, Donner RM: Advances in noninvasive evaluation of congenital anomalies of the thoracic aorta. Radiol Clin North Am 23(4):727–736, 1985
33. Stewart JR, Kincaid O, Edwards J: Atlas of Vascular Rings and Related Malformations of the Aortic Arch System. Springfield, Charles C Thomas, 1964
34. Strife JL, Baumel AS, Dunbar JS: Tracheal compression by the innominate artery in infancy and childhood. Radiology 139:73–75, 1981
35. Tonkin JLD, Holf TR, Moser D, Laster RE Jr: Evaluation of vascular rings with digital subtraction angiography. AJR 142:1287–1291, 1984
36. Yeager SB, Chin AJ, Sanders SP: Two-dimensional echocardiographic diagnosis of pulmonary artery sling in infancy. JACC 7:625–629, 1986

chapter 7

Tracheomalacia

H. Biemann Othersen, Jr., M.D.
Robert M. Filler, M.D.

DEFINITION

Tracheomalacia, recognized and described in the 1950s and 1960s,[2] is the condition in which the structural integrity of the trachea is lost and the cartilaginous rings are not rigid enough to prevent collapse, especially on expiration. Another type of tracheomalacia occurs when the cartilaginous rings do not have the usual horseshoe shape, but are more flattened, thereby allowing the membranous trachea to bulge inward and reduce the size of the airway.[5] The suffix *malacia* denotes "a softening."

In contrast, laryngomalacia may produce symptoms on inspiration, since malacic supraglottic structures such as the epiglottis and aryepiglottic folds may be sucked into the airway on inspiration. Any high airway obstruction, in the presence of tracheomalacia, will produce tracheal collapse on inspiration as well as on expiration (Fig. 7–1).

ETIOLOGY

Tracheomalacia may result from a congenital abnormality in which the entire cartilaginous structure of the airway is abnormal.[7,8] Localized areas of decreased rigidity may also result as the trachea and foregut are formed during embryonal development.[3]

Abnormal pressure on or compression of the cartilaginous rings or a combination of the two causes a gradual constriction or attenuation of the rings in the child with tracheomalacia.[2] For example, an abnormality of development of the great vessels around the trachea produces a vascular ring. The usual unhampered development of the trachea is prevented and, after birth, the constricting blood vessels damage the tracheal wall with pulsatile impingement. Or, in esophageal atresia and tracheoesophageal fistula, the decompressive effect of a distal tracheoesophageal fistula allowing nonphysiologic escape of lung fluid with the loss of tracheal stability is a congenital process.[9] The postoperative tra-

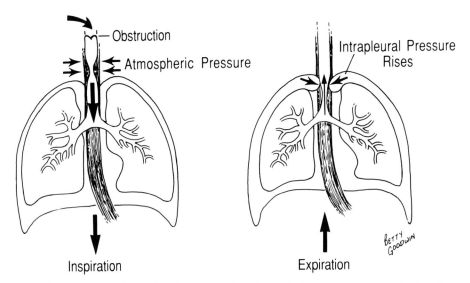

FIGURE 7-1. Airway obstruction from cervical tracheomalacia can occur on inspiration (*left*), whereas intrathoracic tracheomalacia allows obstruction on expiration (*right*).

cheal compression by an enlarged proximal pouch can be considered an acquired process.

PATHOPHYSIOLOGY

Tracheomalacia in the cervical trachea rarely causes significant problems because atmospheric pressure outside the tracheal lumen is the same as inside the tracheal lumen. As noted above in cases of laryngomalacia, however, supraglottic structures may collapse on inspiration as the intratracheal pressure drops and atmospheric pressure pushes the laryngeal tissue as well as air into the glottic lumen. When intrathoracic pressure rises, expiratory collapse of the trachea usually occurs. With a high airway obstruction at the glottis, a soft cervical trachea may collapse on inspiration[23] (see Fig. 7–1).

In the thoracic trachea, negative intrathoracic pressure with inspiration draws air into the lungs as atmospheric pressure is exerted into the airway. On expiration, when the intrathoracic pressure rises, the tracheal wall tends to collapse when it is not rigid (see Fig. 7–1).

Of course, there can be a combination of inspiratory and expiratory obstruction. With compression of the trachea by a large blood vessel the lumen is constricted and the cross-sectional area, on which airflow depends, is reduced. On expiration, when the compressed and softened wall of the trachea further protrudes into the lumen, the obstruction is increased.

CLINICAL FEATURES

Tracheomalacia may be congenital and can occur with no other abnormalities.[7,8] In this situation, structural integrity of the trachea is gradually restored and the child improves with age. There is a diffuse form of tracheomalacia associated with bronchopulmonary dysplasia in small infants. This condition is an entirely

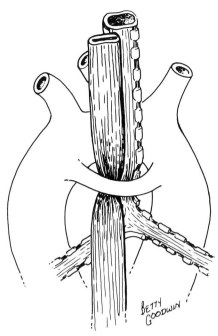

FIGURE 7–2. Both trachea and esophagus are compressed by vascular rings.

different problem and will not be discussed here. Other clinical situations are discussed in the following sections.

Vascular Ring

Any abnormality in the development of the branchial arch vessels may result in a constricting ring around the trachea and esophagus. A confined space is thereby created, and the trachea and esophagus are compressed or restricted. The severity of symptoms depends on the amount of constriction: double aortic arches usually create more difficulties than other rings (Fig. 7–2). When the child swallows, the distending esophagus further compromises the tracheal lumen and increases the obstruction.

Esophageal Atresia and Tracheoesophageal Fistula

The embryonal developmental defect that results in esophageal atresia and tracheoesophageal fistula may also include structural abnormalities of the trachea such as localized tracheomalacia.[21] After repair of the esophagus, the child may develop ''dying spells.'' A less alarming but no less descriptive term for these episodes has been *reflex apnea.* Apnea, cyanosis, and marked bradycardia (usually after feeding) are hallmarks of these ''spells.'' A dilated proximal esophagus appears to be the culprit (Figs. 7–3 and 7–4).

Upon swallowing, esophageal anastomotic constriction causes further distension of the dilated proximal esophagus with increased anterior displacement of

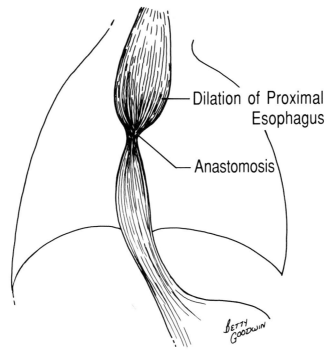

FIGURE 7–3. After repair of esophageal atresia, the proximal esophagus, which is already enlarged, is further dilated by anastomotic stricture.

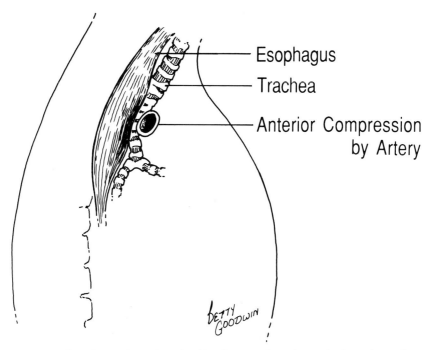

FIGURE 7–4. A lateral view shows how the dilated proximal esophagus displaces the trachea and compresses it against the overlying innominate artery.

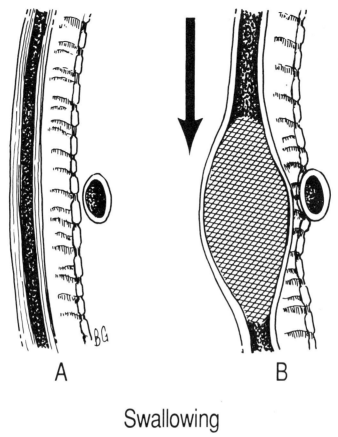

Swallowing

FIGURE 7–5. An enlarged diagram of Figure 7–4 illustrates how the compression is increased by ingestion of a feeding.

the trachea into the innominate artery (Fig. 7–5). The child then becomes apneic and bradycardic, and cardiac arrest may ensue. Because of their suddenness, these episodes were once thought to be due to vagal reflexes.[16] Oxygen monitoring during these attacks, however, has shown that they are associated with hypoxia and may simply be severe hypoxic episodes.[11] Absolute cessation of the "dying spells" after aortopexy further corroborates this theory.[6]

Anomalous Innominate Artery

This condition is still the cause for considerable controversy and concern. Some children do have a developmental defect of the aortic arch whereby the innominate artery arises from the aortic arch in such a manner as to pass over and compress the trachea. Gross and Neuhauser first described this condition and "aortopexy," the operation for its relief.[12]

A report in 1969, however, described 285 patients over a 16-year period with compression of the trachea by the innominate artery.[16] Only 39 (13.7%) had aortopexy performed; the rest were successfully treated medically. It is evident that this syndrome can be overdiagnosed and surgically overtreated.

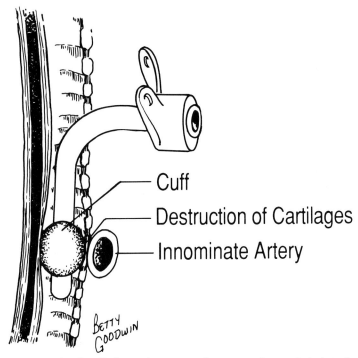

FIGURE 7-6. An inflated cuff of a tracheostomy tube may erode anteriorly into the innominate artery.

Internal Compression

Internal compression of the tracheal wall from cuffed endotracheal or tracheostomy tubes can produce erosion of the cartilaginous rings with tracheomalacia. If protracted, the tracheal cartilaginous structure may be destroyed and the wall perforated (Fig. 7–6). Note that cuffed tubes are rarely required in children because compensation for air leaks around the tube can be made by increasing inspiratory volume.

AIDS TO DIAGNOSIS

Radiographic

Static anteroposterior and lateral radiographs may show airway compression, but a better diagnostic measure is cinefluoroscopy. This technique can demonstrate the dynamics of airway expansion and collapse during inspiration and expiration. With cinefluoroscopy, a small catheter is introduced into the upper esophagus under fluoroscopy. Contrast medium is then injected in order to visualize the effect of swallowing and esophageal distension on the airway.

Endoscopic

Laryngoscopy and rigid bronchoscopy, with the patient anesthetized and breathing spontaneously, will demonstrate directly the distortion and compression of the tracheal lumen. Instead of a circular lumen, the tracheal passage may

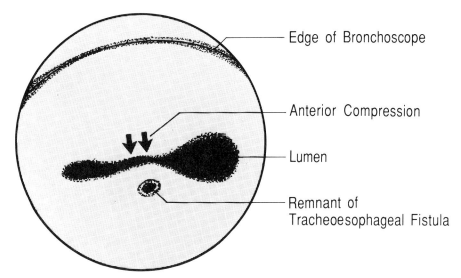

Edge of Bronchoscope

Anterior Compression

Lumen

Remnant of
Tracheoesophageal Fistula

FIGURE 7–7. A bronchoscopic view of the compression of the tracheal lumen by the innominate artery.

appear elliptical and almost slitlike (Fig. 7–7), and pulsation of compressing vessels can be visualized through the tracheal wall. Air exchange should improve when the bronchoscope is passed beyond the area of compression or collapse. Continuous intraoperative monitoring of oxygen saturation is essential, and endoscopy is necessary to the diagnosis.[6,7]

SURGICAL THERAPY

Indications for Operation

With the clinical features described above, episodes of reflex apnea ("dying spells") are so real and frightening to the family and physician that even one such spell is an indication for operation. A recent review of children who underwent aortopexy at Medical University of South Carolina Children's Hospital indicated that young patients who require aortopexy following repair of esophageal atresia uniformly did well and had no further "spells" after operation.[6] Patients who did not have esophageal atresia and who had operation for other causes of tracheomalacia had far less satisfactory results. A review of eight years' experience in Toronto showed similar good results from aortopexy in the treatment of tracheomalacia after repair of esophageal atresia.[4] An earlier review there had shown elimination of "dying spells" by aortopexy.[17] Other authors concur with these findings.[14]

With vascular rings, the operation for division of the constricting vessels should also include retraction and fixation of those vessels. It is thus mandatory to perform endoscopy after correction of a vascular ring to ensure that the tracheal lumen is no longer compressed.

Aortopexy

Aortopexy is the term given to the operation originally described by Gross[12] in which the innominate artery and arch of the aorta are elevated from the trachea

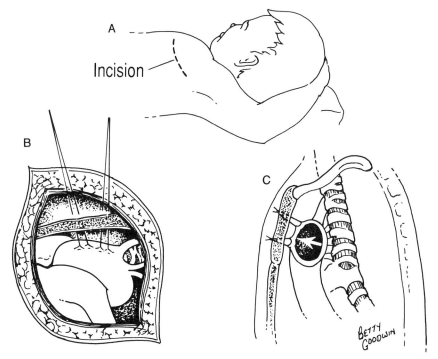

FIGURE 7-8. The operative technique for aortopexy: *A*, anterior left thoracotomy in the third interspace; *B*, sutures placed into the wall of the innominate artery and the aortic arch; *C*, sutures passed through the sternum and tied to elevate the compressing vessels. Tracheal attachments pull the anterior wall of the trachea forward.

and suspended to the sternum. The idea is not to pull the artery away from the trachea, but to elevate the artery in such a manner that the attachments to the tracheal wall produce elevation of the tracheal wall itself.

In performing the operation, the trachea is approached through an anterior left thoracotomy, although a right anterior thoracotomy has also been advocated.[16] Sutures are placed in the wall of compressing vessel (usually the innominate), continuing down onto the arch of the aorta (Fig. 7–8). Care should be taken to ensure that the sutures do not pass into the lumen of the vessel. The sutures can then be either passed through the sternum itself and tied on the ventral surface of the bone or attached to the periosteum on the undersurface of the sternum. Either way the vessel is thus lifted from the trachea, thereby pulling the tracheal wall outward (see Fig. 7–8). It is essential that no dissection between the vessel and the trachea be done. Recently, Applebaum and Woolley[1] described a modification of this procedure using a pericardial flap for suspension of the aortic arch. They found that this modification was satisfactory in elevating the trachea and made the procedure easier to perform.

Internal Stenting

Internal stenting is possible when the tracheomalacic segment can be traversed by a tube. Since endotracheal tubes cannot be left in the larynx indefinitely, a tracheostomy is required. One of us (HBO) has developed a special long tracheostomy tube that can be custom-made in the operating room (as indicated in Fig. 7–9) to pass beyond the area of narrowing and serve as a stent. Other

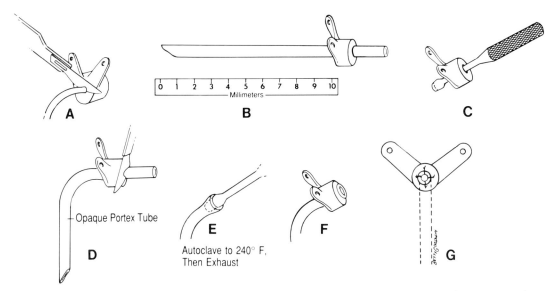

FIGURE 7–9. Details of construction of a custom-made internal tracheal stent. This tube can be made to traverse a low tracheal stricture and is well tolerated for long periods of time.

techniques of construction have been described.[18] It is important to ensure that any external compression has been relieved, such as correction of a vascular ring by division and aortopexy. If an internal stent is placed without correction of a constriction, erosion of the trachea and eventual tracheal stenosis may develop. If the compression has been relieved and the trachea still collapses, the insertion of a tracheostomy stent may allow the tracheal wall to become rigid with time, and eventually the tracheostomy can be removed. Sometimes tracheostomy and continuous positive airway pressure are required for diffuse tracheomalacia.[22]

External Splinting

One of us (RMF) has developed an external splint to be used in those cases of tracheomalacia that cannot be corrected by aortopexy and in those in which the etiology is not vascular compression.[10] This splint has been constructed of Marlex mesh and silicone and has been used in six children, with five excellent long-term results. In one child, the posterior wall of the trachea was somewhat concave but remained stable.[19] The only long-term complication in the group was a collection of serous fluid between the splint and the trachea. Removal of the splint was required, but tracheomalacia did not recur.

The Toronto group developed an animal model for tracheomalacia by creating tracheal defects in pigs.[20] An earlier experimental study had shown no appreciable effect on growth of the trachea when an external prosthetic splint of Silastic and Marlex was utilized.[15] Johnston described external splints using rib grafts in pigs and subsequently in patients.[13]

Tracheoplasty

In some patients with localized tracheomalacia, effective therapy can be accomplished by incising the area of collapse and inserting a rigid piece of cartilage extending to the normal trachea at each end. When the cartilage graft is sutured to adjacent normal trachea, collapse is prevented. (See Chapter 9 for the technique of cartilage tracheoplasty.)

REFERENCES

1. Applebaum H, Woolley MM: Pericardial flap aortopexy for tracheomalacia. J Pediatr Surg 25 (1):30–32, 1990.
2. Baxter JD, Dunbar JS: Tracheomalacia. Ann Otol Rhinol Laryngol 72:1013–1023, 1963.
3. Benjamin B, Cohen D, Glasson M: Tracheomalacia in association with congenital tracheoesophageal fistula. Surgery 79:504–508, 1976.
4. Blair GK, Filler RM, Cohen R: Treatment of tracheomalacia: Eight years' experience. J Pediatr Surg 21:781–785, 1986.
5. Campbell AH, Young IF: Tracheobronchial collapse, a variant of obstructive respiratory disease. Br J Dis Chest 57:174–181, 1963.
6. Clevenger FW, Othersen HB, Smith CD: Relief of tracheal compression by aortopexy. Ann Thorac Surg, in press.
7. Cogbill TH, Moore FA, Accurso FJ, Lilly JR: Primary tracheomalacia. Ann Thorac Surg 35:538–541, 1983.
8. Cox WL Jr, Shaw RR: Congenital chondromalacia of the trachea. J Thorac Cardiovasc Surg 49:1033–1039, 1965.
9. Davies MRQ, Cywes S: The flaccid trachea and tracheoesophageal congenital anomalies. J Pediatr Surg 13(4):363–367, 1978.
10. Filler RM, Buck JR, Bahoric A, et al: Treatment of segmental tracheomalacia and bronchomalacia by implantation of an airway splint. J Pediatr Surg 17:597–603, 1982.
11. Filler RM, Rossello PJ, Lebowitz RL: Life-threatening anoxic spells caused by tracheal compression after repair of esophageal atresia: Correction by surgery. J Pediatr Surg 11:739–748, 1976.
12. Gross RE, Neuhauser EB: Compression of the trachea by an anomalous innominate artery. An operation for its relief. Am J Dis Child 75:570–574, 1948.
13. Johnston MR, Loeber N, Hillyer P, et al: External stent for repair of secondary tracheomalacia. Ann Thorac Surg 30:291–296, 1980.
14. Kiely EM, Spitz L, Brereton R: Management of tracheomalacia by aortopexy. Pediatr Surg Int 2:13–15, 1987.
15. Murphy P, Filler RM, Muraji T, et al: Effect of prosthetic airway splint on the growing trachea. J Pediatr Surg 18:872–878, 1983.
16. Mustard WT, Bayliss CE, Fearon B, et al: Tracheal compression by the innominate artery in children. Ann Thorac Surg 8:312–319, 1969.
17. Schwartz MZ, Filler RM: Tracheal compression as a cause of apnea following repair of tracheoesophageal fistula: Treatment by aortopexy. J Pediatr Surg 15:842–848, 1980.
18. Shapiro RS, Martin WM: Long custom-made plastic tracheostomy tube in severe tracheomalacia. Laryngoscope 91:355–362, 1981.
19. Vinograd I, Filler RM, Bahoric A: Long-term functional results of prosthetic airway splinting in tracheomalacia and bronchomalacia. J Pediatr Surg 22:38–41, 1987.
20. Vinograd I, Filler RM, England SJ, et al: Tracheomalacia. An experimental animal model for a new surgical approach. J Surg Res 42:597–604, 1987.
21. Wailoo MP, Emery JL: The trachea in children with tracheoesophageal fistula. Histopathology 3:329–338, 1979.
22. Wiseman NE, Duncan PG, Cameron CB: Management of tracheobronchomalacia with continuous positive airway pressure. J Pediatr Surg 20:489–493, 1985.
23. Wittenborg MM, Gyepes MT, Crocker D: Tracheal dynamics in infants with respiratory distress, stridor and collapsing trachea. Radiology 88:653–662, 1967.

chapter 8

Injuries of the Airway: Extrinsic and Intrinsic

H. Biemann Othersen, Jr., M.D.

Intubation injuries produced by ill-fitting or irritating endotracheal tubes rank as the most frequent type of injury to the pediatric larynx, trachea, and bronchi.[13] These injuries are seen in children of all ages but are especially prevalent in small, premature infants who are maintained for long periods of time with endotracheal intubation and ventilatory support. In addition, older children with head injuries and complex cardiovascular procedures are routinely managed with long-term endotracheal intubation and respiratory support. Given the circumstances, it is remarkable that there are not more airway injuries than those presently seen.

Children are particularly susceptible to intrinsic airway injuries for the following reasons:

1. The child's trachea is much smaller than that of the adult and thus is more easily obstructed by granulation and scar.
2. Anatomic differences in the pediatric and adult airway invite the unwary physician to insert tubes that are too large for the child's airway. In adults, the smallest part of the airway is the glottis; in children, the lumen is smaller at the cricoid than at the glottis. Thus, in the adult patient, an endotracheal tube that fits easily through the glottis will fit nicely within the rest of the airway. Not so for the child. A tube that fits through the child's glottic opening at the vocal cords may very well be too snug at the cricoid (Fig. 8–1).[13]
3. Laryngotracheal infections such as croup and epiglottitis occur more frequently in children than in adults. Tubes inserted through an inflamed airway may cause pressure necrosis as edema progresses.
4. Congenital stenosis of the airway may be asymptomatic until a respiratory infection (common in small children) further decreases the diameter of the airway by edema. Remember that in the trachea the determinant of airflow

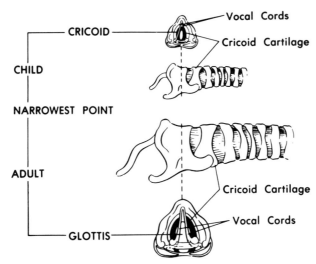

FIGURE 8-1. Difference between adult and pediatric airway. (Reprinted with permission from Othersen HB Jr: Intubation injuries of the trachea in children. Management and prevention. Ann Surg 189:601–606, 1979.)

is the cross-sectional area, which depends upon the square of the radius. Consequently, reduction of the tracheal radius by 10% will result in a reduction of the cross-sectional area by approximately 20%.

5. Some life-threatening conditions such as intrathoracic stenotic lesions and complete tracheal rings are not seen in adults. These problems are either corrected early or the affected children die.

This chapter is concerned only with intrinsic and external injuries to the larynx, trachea, and mainstem bronchi. For a complete treatise on thoracic injuries in children, refer to the chapter on cardiothoracic injuries in *Pediatric Trauma*, edited by Touloukian.[15]

INTERNAL INJURIES

Endotracheal Intubation

By far the greatest number of airway injuries in children are the result of endotracheal intubation. In the past, tubes made of Latex rubber or of the Cole design caused injury as a result of their construction or their design. Most tubes used at present, however, are made of polyvinyl plastic and the material is fairly well tolerated. The clear, plastic tubes remain slightly more rigid than the opaque tubes, which are more difficult to insert.

The size of the endotracheal tube is traditionally the greatest culprit in the production of injury. If the tube is too large or subsequently becomes too large owing to intrinsic tracheal edema, pressure necrosis, ulceration, and eventual scarring will occur. Larger tubes are also less compliant and tend to shift more with head movement and during respiration.[19] Nasotracheal intubation tends to stabilize the tube more, and movement of the tongue and posterior pharynx does not dislodge the tube. A positive pressure ventilator attached to the tube transmits a pistonlike movement, which can be especially damaging if the tube fits too tightly.

Cuffed Endotracheal Tubes

Cooper and Grillo demonstrated that the important factor in the etiology of airway injury is pressure necrosis produced by the inflated cuff of an endotracheal tube.[2] They also produced lesions experimentally and subsequently designed a low-pressure cuff to minimize tracheal injury.[1,5]

Endotracheal tubes with cuffs are not required in children. A cuff will occasionally be necessary in teenagers, but only during acute resuscitation, when it may help to prevent aspiration of regurgitated gastric contents. Because air leaks around the endotracheal tube can easily be compensated for by increasing the volume of inspired air, a cuff should rarely be necessary for ventilatory support.

Tracheostomy Stoma

The use of unyielding metal endotracheal tubes, which cause ulceration at their tips, is unnecessary[14]; polyvinyl and Silastic tubes, which cause little tissue injury, are available (Fig. 8–2). Technique in construction of the tracheostomy, however, is still important. The type of tracheal incision and care of the tracheostomy are essential ingredients for a good result (Fig. 8–3) (see Chapter 15).

Inhalation Injuries

Edema may make an endotracheal tube fit too tightly. Keeping this in mind, refer to the nose as a guide and use an opaque Portex tube one size smaller than normal. Burned children often have inhalation injuries along with their serious cutaneous burns.[10] In a study of adult burn patients, progression of upper airway edema correlated with the severity of cutaneous injury and was increased by intravenous fluids.[8]

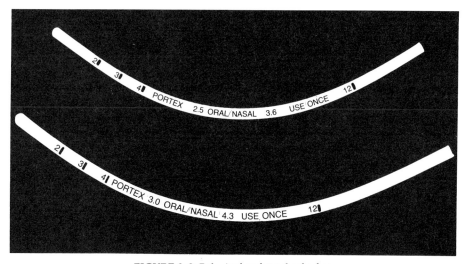

FIGURE 8–2. Polyvinyl endotracheal tubes.

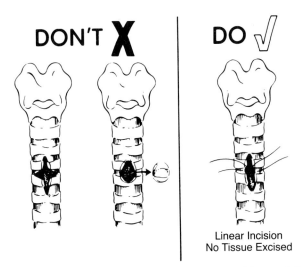

FIGURE 8–3. Two techniques of tracheostomy to be avoided in children and the preferred linear revision. (Reprinted with permission from Othersen HB Jr: Intubation injuries of the trachea in children. Management and prevention. Ann Surg 189:601–606, 1979.)

Respiratory Injuries

It has long been recognized that endotracheal intubation and ventilatory support by a respirator can compound tracheal injury by imparting a shearing force to the tube and increasing tracheal and laryngeal damage.[13] In addition, the new high-frequency ventilators and especially the very high-frequency jet ventilators produce significant mucosal damage near the tip of the endotracheal tube.[11]

EXTERNAL INJURIES

Blunt

A child restrained within a car may be thrown forward into the windshield, and, as a consequence, the neck may hit the dashboard, causing a blunt injury (Fig. 8–4). A child riding a bicycle or motorcycle may sustain a "clothesline" injury, which, in turn, may result in complete transection of the trachea and esophagus without any external evidence of injury to the skin (Fig. 8–5). Note that not only is complete radiographic examination necessary in neck injuries, but endoscopic evaluation of the trachea and esophagus is essential as well.

Most external injuries in small children will be of the blunt variety. The small child has a very pliable chest wall, and the ribs may bend without breaking, thereby imparting the entire force of injury to the underlying airway and lungs. The trachea or bronchi can be ruptured or transected.[9] Possible mechanisms for these ruptures include rapid deceleration with forward swing of the trachea, widening of the transverse diameter of the chest with traction on the carina, and a rapid rise in airway pressure on impact.

It may be more difficult to diagnose blunt injuries than penetrating ones. Although the study was done in adults, Stanley found computed tomography (CT) to be valuable in assessing acute laryngeal injury.[18] In older children with calcified hyoid bones, a lateral film of the neck may show the hyoid to be above the level of the 3rd cervical vertebral body or the greater cornu of the hyoid to

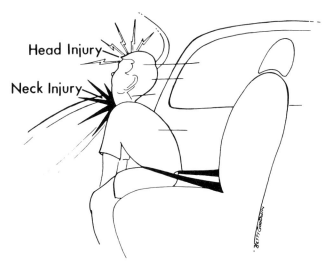

FIGURE 8–4. Mechanism of head airway injury. With a padded dashboard, external evidence of injury is minimal. (Reprinted with permission from Othersen HB Jr: Cardiothoracic injuries. *In* Touloukian RJ (ed): Pediatric Trauma. New York, John Wiley & Sons, 1978, Chap 12.)

be less than 2 cm from the angle of the mandible. With these findings and air in the cervical soft tissues, transection of the trachea should be suspected.[16] Immediate operation may be necessary.

Penetrating

These injuries are uncommon in young children but may be seen in teenagers involved in fights with knives and guns.

The principles in management of airway injuries include the following:
1. Adequate radiographic evaluation and, in any serious blunt or penetrating injury, thorough endoscopic evaluation prior to exploration of the neck.

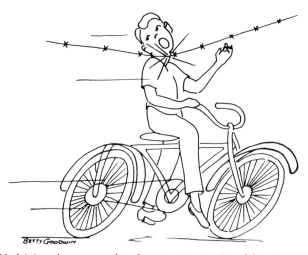

FIGURE 8–5. Neck injury that may produce fracture or transection of the airway with little evidence of skin injury. (Reprinted with permission from Othersen HB Jr: Cardiothoracic injuries. *In* Touloukian RJ (ed): Pediatric Trauma. New York, John Wiley & Sons, 1978, Chap 12.)

2. Primary repair of the injury. Even if a tracheostomy can be established below the injury or endotracheal intubation can be performed, primary repair should be done. THE FIRST OPERATION IS THE BEST OPERATION.

3. Debridement performed with the knowledge that blood supply to the proximal trachea comes from the anterior thyroid artery in the neck.[12,17] Distally, the vascular supply is segmental and enters laterally. *Handle the trachea just as you would the esophagus in esophageal atresia and tracheoesophageal fistula; in other words, be careful with distal mobilization.*

4. When the trachea is completely divided or resection is required, primary repair by either interrupted or continuous absorbable sutures such as Vicryl (polyglycolic acid) or a monofilament suture such as polydioxanone (PDS*). Note that Vicryl sutures are braided, and, although they are absorbable, they can become infected and cause granulation since persistence in the tissue may be prolonged.

The essential elements in the management of airway injuries in children are early recognition and anticipation along with expeditious surgical repair. Since most injuries, internal or external, produce problems by leading to chronic stenosis, it is important to review procedures and techniques that will aid in preventing or ameliorating these strictures of the airway. The techniques developed by Grillo and colleagues[4,7] for the management of surgical procedures on the airway should be reviewed as well as the procedures for prevention of internal injuries and strictures from endotracheal intubation or tracheostomy. The treatment of established strictures is addressed in another chapter.

Grillo and Zannini discussed the factors that are important in dealing with tracheal resections in children.[6] They are:

1. Avoidance of devascularizing the trachea.

2. Avoidance of tension; Grillo found this to be more of a problem in children than in adults, since one-half of the adult trachea can be excised, whereas usually only one-third of the pediatric trachea can be resected without excessive tension.

3. Avoidance of a foreign body, such as a tube, that passes through the anastomosis. Unfortunately, this may be unavoidable in very small infants.

PREVENTION OF STENOSIS

Most internal tracheal injuries are preventable when endotracheal tubes are properly inserted and cared for. Tubes should not fit tightly within the trachea. The external naris of the child can be used as a rough guide to proper tube size (Fig. 8–6). Any tube that passes through the nose without deforming the naris is usually accepted by the trachea. Clear polyvinyl tubes are satisfactory acutely, but for long-term intubation we prefer the opaque polyvinyl tubes (Portex), which tend to soften slightly at body temperature and, as a result, conform to the larynx and trachea (see Fig. 8–2).

A serious, preventable injury to the trachea may be produced by the inflated cuff of an endotracheal or tracheostomy tube. The site of necrosis is often too low within the trachea to be relieved by tracheostomy, and treatment in these cases is difficult. Despite the fact that low-pressure cuffs have been developed to help eliminate this problem,[5] there are actually very few indications for the use of cuffed tubes in children. Even with the tube attached to a respirator, a

---

*Ethicon Inc., Somerville, NJ.

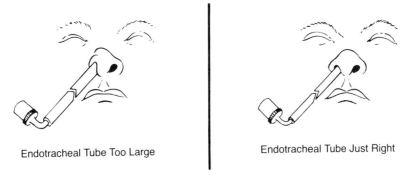

Endotracheal Tube Too Large   Endotracheal Tube Just Right

FIGURE 8–6. An endotracheal tube should fit through the external naris without deforming it.

slight air leak around the tube is desirable because it indicates that the tube does not fit too tightly. Such leaks can be easily compensated for by increasing the tidal volume of the respirator.

Endotracheal intubation is much easier to maintain than tracheostomy in infants under 6 months of age. It is relatively easy, although sedation and muscle relaxants may be required, to restrain the head of these small infants and thereby prevent the shearing action produced by movement of the tube within the trachea.

INDICATIONS FOR TRACHEOSTOMY

The sheer volume of literature on the subject reflects the continuing concern over prolonged endotracheal intubation versus tracheostomy in children. Because complications are often associated with tracheostomy, especially when it is performed in very small infants, we have proposed the following recommendations (see Table 4–2):
1. Prolonged endotracheal intubation is well tolerated and may be managed more effectively than tracheostomy in infants ranging from birth to 6 months of age.
2. In the presence of severe inflammatory glottic and tracheal disease, endotracheal intubation should be performed and maintained only long enough for tracheostomy to be accomplished. Edema in the area of the cricoid may cause pressure against the tube with resultant necrosis.
3. Tracheostomy should be considered in a child over 6 months of age who requires endotracheal intubation for longer than 10 to 14 days.
4. Tracheostomy should be considered in a child over 6 months of age who requires respirator support for longer than 7 to 10 days.
   THE BEST TREATMENT OF AIRWAY INJURIES IN CHILDREN IS AWARENESS AND PREVENTION.

REFERENCES

1. Cooper JD, Grillo HC: Experimental production and prevention of injury due to cuffed tracheal tubes. Surg Gynecol Obstet 129:1235, 1969
2. Cooper JD, Grillo HC: The evolution of tracheal injury due to ventilatory assistance through cuffed tubes: A pathologic study. Ann Surg 169:334, 1969
3. de la Rocha AG: Traumatic rupture of the tracheobronchial tree. Can J Surg 28(1):68–71, 1985

4. Grillo HC: Notes on the windpipe. Ann Thorac Surg 47:9–26, 1989
5. Grillo HC, Cooper JD, Geffin B, Pontoppidan H: A low-pressure cuff for tracheostomy tubes to minimalize tracheal injury. J Thorac Cardiovasc Surg 62:898, 1971
6. Grillo HC, Zannini P: Management of obstructive tracheal disease in children. J Pediatr Surg 19:414, 1984
7. Grillo HC, Zannini P, Michelassi F: Complications of tracheal reconstruction. J Thorac Cardiovasc Surg 91:322–328, 1986
8. Haponik EF, Meyers DA, Munster AM, Smith PL, Britt EJ, Wise RA, Bleecker ER: Acute upper airway injury in burn patients. Am Rev Respir Dis 135(2):360–366, 1987
9. Hughes MJ, Hayes OW, Guertin SR, McGillicuddy, JE: Traumatic rupture of right mainstem bronchus in a child. J Emerg Med 4(6):443–447, 1986
10. Judkins KC, Brander WL: Respiratory injury in children: The histology of healing. Burns Incl Therm Inj 12(5):357–359, 1986
11. Mammel MC, Ophoven JP, Lewallen PK, Gordon MJ, Sutton MC, Boros SJ: High-frequency ventilation and tracheal injuries. Pediatrics 77(4):608–613, 1986
12. Miura T, Grillo HC: The contribution of the inferior thyroid artery to the blood supply of the human trachea. Surg Gynecol Obstet 123:99, 1966
13. Othersen HB Jr: Intubation injuries of the trachea in children. Management and prevention. Ann Surg 189:601–606, 1979
14. Othersen HB Jr: Trachea, lungs, pleural cavity. *In* Welch K (ed): Complications in Pediatric Surgery. Philadelphia, W.B. Saunders Co., 1982
15. Othersen HB Jr: Cardiothoracic injuries. *In* Touloukian RJ (ed): Pediatric Trauma. New York, John Wiley & Sons, 1978, Chap 12
16. Polansley A, Resnick D, Sofferman RA, Davidson TM: Hyoid bone elevation: A sign of tracheal transection. Radiol 150:117–120, 1984
17. Salassa JR, Pearson BW, Payne WS: Gross and microscopical blood supply of the trachea. Ann Thorac Surg 24:100, 1977
18. Stanley RB Jr: Value of computed tomography in management of acute laryngeal injury. J Trauma 24(4):359–362, 1984
19. Whitel R: A study of endotracheal tube injury to the subglottis. Laryngoscope 95:1216–1219, 1985

part 3

The Laryngotracheoplasties

chapter 9

Cricoid Split and Cartilage Tracheoplasty

Charles M. Myer III, M.D.
Robin T. Cotton, M.D.

MANAGEMENT OF SUBGLOTTIC STENOSIS IN INFANTS AND CHILDREN

The management of subglottic stenosis in infants and children continues to evolve. This chapter explores the surgical options currently utilized at our institution and the rationale involved in the choice of these reconstructive procedures.

Once a child with a potential subglottic stenosis is identified, microlaryngoscopy and bronchoscopy are performed in the operating room. If the child does not have an endotracheal tube in place, a flexible laryngoscopy is performed before rigid endoscopy in an effort to ascertain vocal cord mobility as well as to examine the subglottis. Rigid endoscopy is usually necessary to evaluate the subglottic area.

During the endoscopic procedure, one must evaluate carefully all areas of the larynx and trachea. Specifically, one must carefully delineate the region of narrowing, taking care to identify whether the stenosis is located anteriorly, laterally, posteriorly, or in some combination thereof. This point is especially important in surgical planning, since an isolated anterior subglottic stenosis is handled differently than a lateral or posterior stenosis.

In general, isolated anterior subglottic stenoses can be managed effectively with an anterior cricoid split procedure in the neonate or very young infant, whereas an autogenous costal cartilage reconstruction is usually utilized in the older child. Children, however, who present with circumferential, lateral, or posterior stenosis are treated differently. In these patients, a laryngofissure is frequently combined with division of the posterior cricoid lamina and placement of a stent. In some of these patients, autogenous costal cartilage is placed posteriorly between the divided segments of the cricoid. In other patients, lateral cricoid incisions are used to further increase the size of the lumen. A stent is placed in almost all patients who have an element of glottic stenosis.[1,3,4]

ANTERIOR CRICOID SPLIT PROCEDURE

Although originally developed as an alternative to tracheostomy in neonates with subglottic stenosis,[6] the anterior cricoid split procedure is now an acceptable form of therapy for mild to moderate laryngeal stenosis in both infants and children and does not have a definable upper age limit. It should be performed only after endoscopic confirmation of anterior glottic or subglottic narrowing. The procedure should be performed through an open surgical technique and not in a percutaneous fashion. It is generally not performed unless the child has failed extubation on several occasions because of laryngeal abnormalities.

Other criteria that should be met before the performance of an anterior cricoid split procedure include the following:

Patient weight greater than 1500 gm
No assisted ventilation for 10 days before the procedure
Supplemental oxygen requirement less than 35%
No congestive heart failure for 1 month before the procedure
No acute upper or lower respiratory tract infection at the time of operation
No antihypertensive medication for 10 days before the procedure

At the time of the initial endoscopic examination, secondary lesions of the larynx and trachea should be noted since they may prevent success of an anterior cricoid split procedure and influence the physician to perform a tracheostomy instead. Correction of the secondary problem before attempted extubation, however, may preclude the necessity of an anterior cricoid split procedure or, alternatively, may allow the anterior cricoid split procedure to be successful. Mobility of the vocal cords and choanal patency should also be assessed before performing an anterior cricoid split procedure.

The anterior cricoid split procedure is performed in the operating room with the patient positioned on a shoulder roll (Fig. 9–1A). Airway control is maintained with either a ventilating bronchoscope or an endotracheal tube. After injection of a local anesthetic, a horizontal skin incision is made over the cricoid to expose the cricoid cartilage, the lower portion of the thyroid cartilage, and the upper trachea. A combination of sharp and blunt dissection is then used to skeletonize the larynx and upper trachea (Fig. 9–1B), and a single vertical incision is made through the anterior cartilaginous ring of the cricoid and its underlying mucosa. The incision is extended inferiorly through the upper two tracheal rings and superiorly through the lower portion of the thyroid cartilage, generally stopping just below the vocal cords (Fig. 9–1C). If the stenosis involves the glottis, the incision is extended up through the vocal cords.

Once the incision is made, the patient is intubated with an appropriately sized endotracheal tube to serve as a stent (Fig. 9–1D). In general, patients who weigh 1500 to 2000 gm are given a 3.0-mm tube, whereas those who weigh 2000 to 2500 gm have a 3.5-mm tube placed. A 4.0-mm tube is reserved for children weighing 2500 to 3000 gm. Retention sutures of 4-0 Prolene are placed on each side of the cricoid incision. These sutures are useful during the postoperative period if the endotracheal tube becomes dislodged and cannot be reinserted

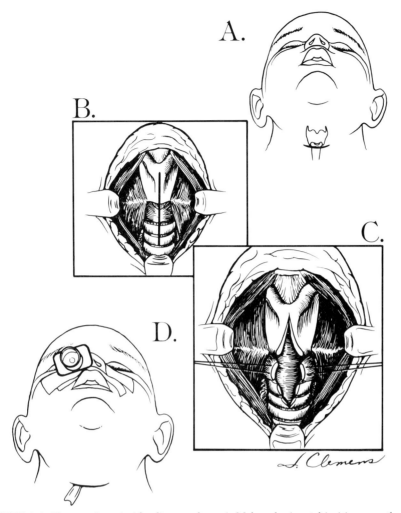

FIGURE 9–1. The anterior cricoid split procedure. *A,* Make a horizontal incision over the cricoid cartilage. *B,* Utilize a combination of sharp and blunt dissection to expose the larynx and upper trachea. *C,* Split the lower portion of the thyroid cartilage, the cricoid cartilage, and upper tracheal rings. *D,* Close the wound loosely over a drain with the airway stented by a nasotracheal tube.

from above. The traction sutures can then be pulled laterally and a tracheostomy tube inserted. The wound is closed loosely around an elastic band drain, which is left in place for 24 to 48 hours.

Patients weighing less than 2500 gm at the time of the procedure generally have a stent placed for approximately 14 days. Patients who weigh more than 2500 gm have their stent in place for 7 days. Dexamethasone sodium phosphate (1 mg/kg/day) in divided doses is administered intravenously, orally, or via nasogastric tube for 24 hours before extubation and for 4 days following extubation. Steroid treatment is discontinued if malignant hypertension develops.

After extubation, patients receive humidified air and racemic epinephrine treatment as needed. Chest physiotherapy and suctioning are also performed when necessary. The patient receives nothing by mouth for 24 hours after extubation. Should postextubation airway obstruction develop, the child is reintubated with a 3.0-mm endotracheal tube. An effort is made to extubate the patient after an additional period of intubation, and, if this fails, endoscopy is performed again to assess the need for a repeat anterior cricoid split procedure or other surgical intervention (such as the removal of tracheal granulation tissue or a tracheostomy).

Under no circumstances should this procedure be performed in a facility unable to deal with critically ill infants. Expert nursing care and support from an intensive care physician are essential to prevent accidental extubation or plugging of the endotracheal tube. Sedation and, occasionally, paralysis with assisted ventilation may be necessary. Although the retention sutures placed at the initial procedure may allow prompt reinsertion of an endotracheal or tracheostomy tube through the neck during an emergency situation, the health care team's goal should be to *prevent* a catastrophic situation, not to remedy it.[2,3,5]

OPEN SURGICAL REPAIR

In the older child with subglottic stenosis, an anterior cricoid split procedure may not provide enough enlargement of the lumen to allow tracheostomy removal. Open reconstruction is generally recommended when the stenosis is greater than 70%. But before surgical repair, vocal cord mobility must be assured via flexible laryngoscopy, and the presence of posterior glottic or subglottic stenosis should be evaluated carefully during rigid endoscopy. Failure to recognize mobility problems may lead to a poor surgical result.

The operative goal should be to provide a satisfactory airway for early decannulation while minimizing any detrimental effects on the voice. Patients who demonstrate incompetence of the gastroesophageal junction with gastroesophageal reflux should be considered for antireflux therapy before corrective laryngeal surgery is undertaken. Untreated reflux frequently leads to excessive granulation tissue in the glottis and subglottis following surgical repair. Laryngoplasty is also contraindicated in a patient in whom a tracheostomy would still be necessary following repair of laryngeal stenosis. Patients, however, with severe stenosis who are on a ventilator may choose to have reconstructive surgery performed in an effort to improve phonation and the ability to communicate. Although most patients weigh more than 10 kg at the time of surgery, there is no lower limit that would preclude intervention.

Several operative approaches are generally used in patients with a fibrous subglottic stenosis without significant loss of cartilaginous support. When the stenosis is limited to the anterior subglottis, an anterior autogenous costal cartilage graft is appropriate. When the stenosis is more circumferential, the cricoid may be divided anteriorly, posteriorly, and possibly laterally, and a stent placed. When the stenosis extends into the glottis, placement of a stent is essential. In selected patients with an upper tracheal stenosis, a segmental resection of the trachea with an end-to-end anastomosis may be successful. In these cases, a suprahyoid release may be necessary to prevent anastomotic tension.[1,3,4]

AUTOGENOUS COSTAL CARTILAGE RECONSTRUCTION

Following induction of general anesthesia through an existing tracheostomy, microlaryngoscopy and bronchoscopy are performed to confirm the site of ste-

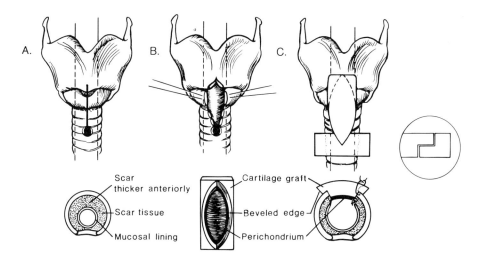

Scar thicker anteriorly
Scar tissue
Mucosal lining

Cartilage graft
Beveled edge
Perichondrium

Perichondrium must face internally

FIGURE 9–2. An autogenous costal cartilage graft reconstruction. *A,* Expose the larynx and upper trachea. *B,* Incise the aforementioned region, remaining superior to the tracheostomy stoma if the stenosis does not involve this site. *C,* Sew the costal cartilage to the incised edges of the larynx and trachea, placing the perichondrium internally.

nosis and proposed surgical repair. The patient is placed in the supine position with the neck hyperextended using a shoulder bolster. Costal cartilage is generally removed from a rib below the skin incision in the inframammary crease. The perichondrium on the anterior aspect of the rib is included, but the posterior perichondrium is left in situ against the pleura. The wound is closed in layers over a small Penrose drain, which is removed after approximately 24 hours.

The larynx is exposed via a U-shaped skin incision over the cricoid cartilage and the superior aspect of the stoma (Fig. 9–2A). The cricoid cartilage is split vertically in the midline through the intraluminal scar and underlying mucosa to enter the tracheal lumen (Fig. 9–2B). Care is taken to extend the incision superiorly in the midline of the thyroid cartilage to a point just below the anterior commissure. The incision is then extended inferiorly for several rings. Should the stenosis reach to the level of the tracheostomy, the incision must extend this far as well. No attempt is made to remove scar tissue.

The costal cartilage graft is then shaped in an elliptical fashion with flanges extending at each end to lie across the cut margin of the thyroid cartilage superiorly and the tracheal wall inferiorly. This prevents accidental dislodgement of the graft into the tracheal lumen. The largest graft that can be placed easily between the cut edges of the thyroid, cricoid, and tracheal cartilages is used with the perichondrial surface facing the lumen. The graft is sewn into position with a 4-0 Vicryl suture in an extramucosal mattress fashion (Fig. 9–2C). The wound is then closed in layers over a small Penrose drain, which is left in place for several days. Before leaving the operating room, a 0° telescope is used to assess the position of the graft and the increase in subglottic and upper tracheal lumen site. If the results are unsatisfactory, the graft must be repositioned.

The child is generally discharged from the hospital 5 days after surgery and endoscopy is performed approximately 6 weeks later. If the increase in lumen size is satisfactory, the decannulation process may begin.[1,3,4,8]

COMBINED LARYNGOFISSURE AND DIVISION OF POSTERIOR CRICOID LAMINA

After the induction of general anesthesia, microlaryngoscopy and bronchoscopy are performed to evaluate the degree of laryngeal and tracheal scarring and the appropriateness of the planned surgical procedure. A U-shaped incision is made that incorporates the upper portion of the stoma (Fig. 9–3A). The larynx and trachea are exposed, and a midline anterior incision extending from the superior thyroid notch to the tracheostomy site is made in the larynx and upper trachea (Fig. 9–3B). The posterior cricoid lamina and scar are injected with 1% Xylocaine with 1/100,000 epinephrine in the posterior scar, and the posterior lamina of the cricoid is divided (Fig. 9–3C). Care must be taken to stay in the midline without entering the hypopharynx or upper cervical esophagus. In cases of

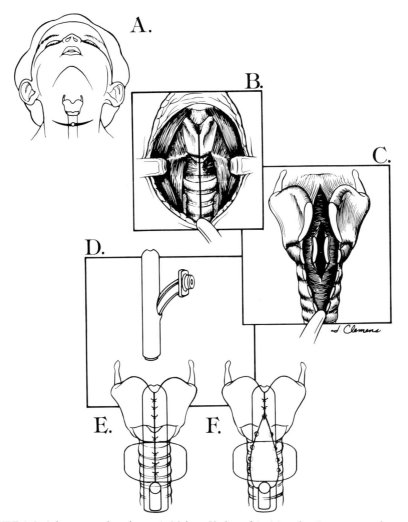

FIGURE 9–3. A laryngotracheoplasty. *A,* Make a U-shaped incision that incorporates the tracheostomy stoma. *B,* Expose the larynx and upper trachea. *C,* Divide the larynx anteriorly and, if necessary, posteriorly (and possibly place a graft). *D,* Place an Aboulker stent with a metal tracheostomy tube incorporated into the stent. *E,* Close the anterior incision primarily. *F,* Alternatively, place a costal cartilage graft.

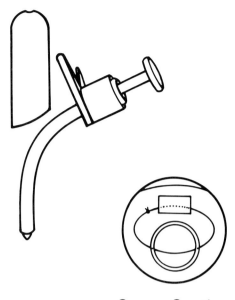

Cross Section

FIGURE 9–4. Tracheostomy tube placed below the Aboulker stent.

severe stenosis or where there are lateral shelves, lateral cricoid incisions may also be necessary.

The posterior incision is extended superiorly into the interarytenoid area (as far as the interarytenoid muscle) and inferiorly into the membranous tracheo-esophageal septum approximately 1 cm below the lower border of the cricoid. The interarytenoid muscle is not divided unless it is found to be fibrosed. In most cases, no posterior graft is placed. When there is an isolated posterior sub-glottic stenosis, however, placement of an autogenous costal cartilage graft between the distracted edges of the posterior cricoid lamina is appropriate.

An Aboulker Teflon stent is inserted to maintain separation of the ends of the cricoid cartilage (Fig. 9–3D) and the tracheal incision closed (Fig. 9–3E and F). The size of the stent is determined by which size tube fits comfortably into the lower tracheal segment. When the stent is to be left for a brief period of time, it is placed above the tracheostomy tube and anchored by sutures through the thyroid cartilage (Fig. 9–4). In cases of severe stenosis, however, the stent is left for up to 12 months and a Holinger-style metal tracheostomy tube is placed into the stent and wired in position with a figure-of-eight 22-gauge wire suture (Fig. 9–5). Upper placement of the stent, which should open just above the vocal cords, is crucial. This position must be confirmed endoscopically before closure of the airway, and the stent should be repositioned if necessary.

In cases of severe stenosis, it may not be possible to close the anterior laryngotracheal fissure. Autogenous cartilage grafting is then necessary in addition to the placement of a stent (see Fig. 9–3F). In such circumstances, the stent is generally left for a prolonged period of time.

As mentioned previously, the stent is left in place for a variable period of time depending on the severity of the stenosis. Care must be taken during the removal of the stent to ensure that it not be broken. This is especially important when the stent and the tracheostomy tube are wired together. Following

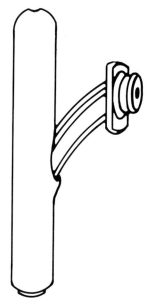

FIGURE 9-5. Aboulker stent with metal tracheostomy tube.

removal of the stent, an appropriately sized tracheostomy tube is placed into the stoma.

For approximately 2 weeks, the child receives inhalational dexamethasone sodium phosphate (1 mg/kg/day) in divided doses, with a maximum of 20 mg/day administered. At this time, another rigid endoscopy is performed and the decannulation process is begun if the lumen is satisfactory. If there is a residual stenosis, either endoscopic or open surgical repair should be considered.[1,3,4,7]

REFERENCES

1. Cotton RT: Pediatric laryngotracheal stenosis. J Pediatr Surg 19:699–704, 1984
2. Cotton RT: Prevention and management of laryngeal stenosis in infants and children. J Pediatr Surg 20:845–851, 1985
3. Cotton RT: The management and prevention of subglottic stenosis in infants and children. Adv Otolaryngol Head Neck Surg 1:241–260, 1987
4. Cotton RT, Myer CM III: Contemporary surgical management of laryngeal stenosis in children. Am J Otolaryngol 5:360–368, 1984
5. Cotton RT, Myer CM III, Bratcher GO, et al: Anterior cricoid split, 1977–1987. Evolution of a technique. Arch Otolaryngol Head Neck Surg 114:1300–1302, 1988
6. Cotton RT, Seid AB: Management of the extubation problem in the premature child. Anterior cricoid split as an alternative to tracheotomy. Ann Otol Rhinol Laryngol 89:508–511, 1980
7. Gray S, Miller R, Myer CM III, et al: Ajunctive measures for successful laryngotracheal reconstruction. Ann Otol Rhinol Laryngol 96:509–513, 1987
8. Zalzal GH, Cotton RT: A new way of carving cartilage grafts to avoid prolapse into the tracheal lumen when used in subglottic reconstruction. Laryngoscope 96:1039, 1986

chapter 10

Endotracheal Cryotherapy for Airway Strictures

Bradley M. Rodgers, M.D.
Eugene D. McGahren, M.D.

Cryotherapy is defined as the use of cold for therapeutic purposes. Although the term became popular in 1907 after Pusey's report on the treatment of skin lesions with carbon dioxide, the therapeutic value of cold has long been recognized.[2,12]

As early as 3500 B.C., the Egyptians used cold to treat fractures and other battle wounds. Thousands of years later, in the 19th century, the surgeon to Napoleon Bonaparte noted that amputations could be carried out with little pain if the diseased or injured limb was first cooled in snow. Arnott, in 1851, was the first physician to utilize the cytotoxic properties of cold when he employed a salt-ice mixture to eradicate skin tumors.[8,16,18] Since that time, agents such as carbon dioxide snow, ether spray, liquid nitrogen, and various refrigerant gases have found a variety of uses in dermatology, ophthalmology, gynecology, neurosurgery, otolaryngology, and general surgery.

A significant breakthrough in the field of cryosurgery occurred in 1961 when Cooper and Lee developed a closed cryogenic system. Using liquid nitrogen as a coolant, they were able to achieve temperatures as low as $-196°C$. The critical component of their system was a probe that allowed selective destruction of undesired tissues. They used the system in the treatment of patients with Parkinson's disease by producing cryodestruction of the basal ganglion.[5]

Neel and Sanderson and their coworkers adapted the principle of cryotherapy to the treatment of obstructing tumors of the airway and reported their findings in the early 1970s.[4,7,11,15] Soon thereafter, in 1978, Rodgers and Talbert reported the clinical application of cryotherapy in the treatment of obstructing lesions of the airway in infants and children.[14] Clinical observations of patients in whom superficial neoplasms have been treated by cryotherapy indicate a rapid regeneration of the epithelium following tumor destruction and a striking lack of fibrous tissue deposition in the affected area. These healing properties associated with cryotherapy have rendered the technique particularly attractive for treatment of lesions of the airway.

PHYSIOLOGY

The mechanism of tissue destruction as a result of cryotherapy is complex and involves at least three phases. The first phase is characterized by cell injury and death during the freeze-thaw cycle. During this period, extracellular and intracellular ice crystals form, resulting in an increased intracellular electrolyte concentration, cellular dehydration, and, ultimately, cellular collapse with denaturation of membrane lipoproteins. Cellular death, for which temperatures of at least −30°C are necessary, is enhanced by a rapid cooling phase followed by a slow thaw. Repetitive freeze-thaw cycles produce an even greater degree of cellular death.[6,10,16]

The second phase of tissue destruction occurs after thawing. At that time, stasis and thrombosis of the microcirculation take place, the result being an area of ischemic tissue.[6,10,16,19]

The third and final phase of tissue destruction by cryotherapy is less defined. It appears that cryotherapy may stimulate an immune response toward the frozen tissue. This reaction perhaps results from a release of antigenic material during cellular disruption. An immune response as a result of cryotherapy has been noted in the treatment of certain malignant tumors and may have important therapeutic implications.[6,10]

EQUIPMENT

A cryoprobe* has been designed specifically for the treatment of airway strictures in infants and children. Measuring 41 cm in length and 3 mm in outside diameter, the cryoprobe may be passed through infant laryngoscopes and bronchoscopes.[13] It is angled at the handle to allow direct visualization down the shaft, and the entire instrument, except for the distal 1 cm, is insulated to prevent freezing of more proximal tissues. Using nitrous oxide as a coolant while relying upon the Joule-Thompson effect (the cooling of gases on sudden expansion), the cryoprobe is able to reach a temperature of −80°C within seconds of activation. The flow of gases through the instrument is activated by a foot pedal connected to a console and regulated by a pressure gauge on the same console. The temperature of the tip of the cryoprobe is monitored by an internal thermocouple and displayed on a second gauge atop the console (Fig. 10–1).

Insertion of a tracheostomy prior to cryotherapy is advised for most infants and for older patients with severe strictures; without the tracheostomy, the edema caused by cryotherapy may precipitate postoperative airway compromise.

Visualization of the airway stricture is achieved under general anesthesia with either a suspension laryngoscope, which is used for glottic and subglottic lesions, or a rigid, ventilating bronchoscope, which is used for more distal

*Frigitronics of Connecticut, Inc., Shelton, CT.

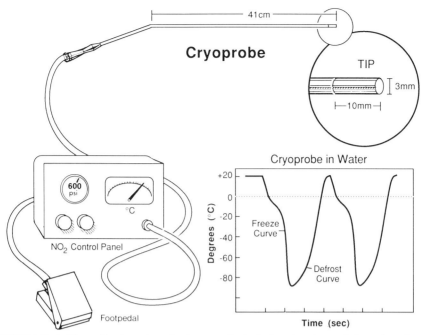

FIGURE 10–1. The pediatric endotracheal cryoprobe is designed to be used through endoscopes with diameters of 3 mm or larger. The flow of nitrous oxide is regulated by a control panel that also records the temperature at the tip of the cryoprobe. The uninsulated tip of the cryoprobe reaches temperatures of $-80°C$ within seconds of the activation of gas flow.

lesions (Fig. 10–2). If the suspension laryngoscope is used, ventilation is maintained by intermittently passing a small endotracheal tube into the upper airway. Before beginning cryotherapy, bronchoscopic surveillance of the distal airway should be performed to identify associated abnormalities. In so doing, particular attention should be directed toward the extent of the lesion and the presence of tracheomalacia in the region of the stricture.

To begin cryotherapy, the cryoprobe is introduced into the airway through the endoscope, and the side of its uninsulated tip is placed against the stricture. The pressure of the nitrous oxide is set at maximum level (600 PSI) on the console, and the flow of gas is initiated with the foot pedal. Within seconds, the temperature at the tip of the probe should reach $0°C$; when this occurs, the probe should be firmly affixed to the stricture. Within another 15 to 20 seconds, the temperature at the tip should drop to $-60°C$. At this point, cryotherapy is measured for 45 to 90 seconds, the duration of the therapy depending upon the severity of the stricture. During this interval, the temperature of the cryoprobe should drift to $-80°C$. If the temperature fails to drop from $-60°C$, one of two situations exists: either the tip of the probe is touching the bronchoscope or the nitrous oxide tanks have lost pressure.

At $-80°C$, a small ball of ice should form around the tip of the cryoprobe and incorporate a portion of the stricture. At the completion of the freeze, the flow of nitrous oxide is stopped and a spontaneous thaw is allowed. At $0°C$, the probe should release from the frozen area, leaving a ball of ice approximately 7 to 10 mm in diameter with a central indentation. At this point, endoscopic biopsy forceps are used for resection of the frozen area, a procedure that should be performed rapidly, before complete thawing is achieved. Bleeding during

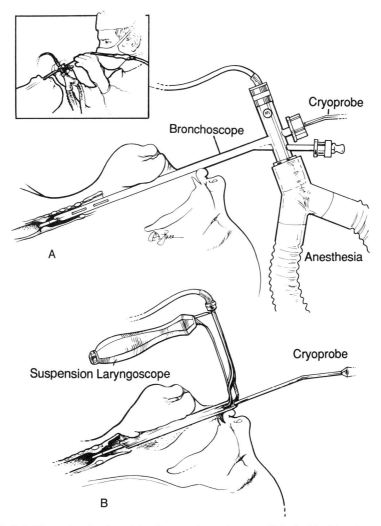

FIGURE 10–2. Direct visualization of the airway stricture is accomplished with either the operating bronchoscope (*A*) or the suspension laryngoscope (*B*). The choice of instrument depends on the location of the stricture in the airway. Careful assessment of the distal tracheal bronchial tree should be accomplished either before or immediately after cryotherapy.

resection is minimal as a result of vasospasm induced by cryotherapy; as the tissue continues to warm, however, slight surface bleeding may occur.

Treatment of approximately 180 degrees of the circumference of the airway often necessitates repeated applications of the cryoprobe to the stricture. We have not recommended any single attempt at endoscopic cryosection extending beyond 270 degrees of the circumference of the airway because of the degree of edema induced.

Because it is difficult at times to resect all of the stricture with the biopsy forceps, a small amount of tissue will occasionally remain following cryotherapy. This residual tissue may be refrozen with the cryoprobe and merely allowed to slough in the 3 or 4 days following cryotherapy. When the maximal amount of tissue has been resected, triamcinolone (40 mg/cc) is injected submucosally into the treated area (Fig. 10–3). The airway is then dilated with Jackson dilators as a means of calibrating the lumen size and forcing the steroids into the submu-

Stricture in Sagittal Section   Stricture Viewed through Scope

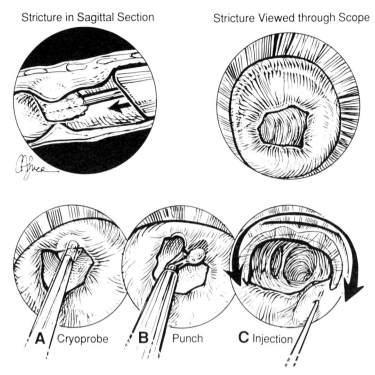

FIGURE 10–3. *A,* After the stricture has been adequately visualized, the tip of the cryoprobe is placed against the most severe area of stricture and the flow of gas is activated. *B,* Following the freeze, a ball of ice forms in the area of application. The ball and the frozen area are then immediately resected with the biopsy forceps. The cryoprobe is then repeatedly applied to the lesion until approximately 180 degrees of the strictured area has been resected. *C,* The submucosal tissues in this region are then injected with triamcinolone.

cosal tissues. We have not employed endotracheal stenting following cryotherapy in the past 12 years; stents were used, however, in some of the earlier patients in our experience.

Most patients experience very little discomfort following cryotherapy. Many have a low-grade fever for 48 hours, and most will experience a productive cough for several days. Patients without a protecting tracheostomy may, however, suffer symptoms of airway obstruction possibly caused by the edema that routinely results from this modality. Systemic steroids have then been used in this setting.

Within 3 to 5 days following cryotherapy, there is a slough of the residual superficial mucosa, and patients may notice mild hemoptysis and a significant increase in the production of mucus. Repeat bronchoscopic evaluation of the airway should be performed within 6 to 12 weeks of the date of therapy, depending on the clinical circumstance. Repeated applications of cryotherapy may then be performed if necessary.

INDICATIONS

The principal indications for endotracheal cryotherapy in the pediatric population are congenital or acquired strictures of the airway. In addition, a small number of children with airway hemangiomas or various airway tumors have been successfully treated with cryotherapy (Table 10–1).[1,3,9]

TABLE 10-1. Endotracheal Cryotherapy in Children

	Strictures			
	Subglottic	*Trachea*	*Mainstem*	**Tumors**
No. patients	20	11	2	3
Age	6 mo–20 yr	1–20 yr	6 mo–1 yr	1–9 yr
Treatments	2.5	2.0	2.0	1.5
Extubated (%)	13/20 (65)	11/11 (100)	1/2 (50)	3/3 (100)
Deaths	4	0	1	0

Between July 1976 and June 1987, we treated 20 children under the age of 20 with strictures of the subglottic airway. Seven of these strictures were considered congenital and the remainder acquired. The ages of the patients at the time of cryotherapy ranged from 6 months to 20 years. All patients had previously been treated with repeated airway dilatations with no success; none, however, had received laser therapy. There were four deaths in the group, three of which were caused by severe associated cardiac anomalies. A fourth patient died at home of a presumed tracheostomy mishap during a course of cryotherapy for a subglottic web. On the basis of our experience with the three infants with severe cardiac lesions, we now recommend simple dilatation of these strictures for the 1st year of life and the commencement of cryotherapy thereafter. Of the surviving 16 patients, 13 (81%) had successful extubation and required an average of 2.5 (range 2 to 4) cryosurgical resections. Repeated cryotherapy has been unsuccessful in relieving subglottic strictures in three patients, and they await more extensive laryngeal procedures.

In the same span of time, we treated 11 patients with cryotherapy for strictures of the distal trachea (see Table 10–1). The age range in this group was from 1 to 20 years. Five of these lesions were secondary to endotracheal intubation, one was secondary to a tracheal resection for trauma, and one was caused by accidental hanging. The remainder were strictures at a tracheostomy stoma. In all of these cases, the strictures have been relieved by cryotherapy with an average of two applications (range 1 to 4), and the patients with tracheostomies have been extubated. In one patient, however, an area of tracheomalacia in the region of the acquired stricture necessitated tracheal resection before successful extubation.

Two cases of strictures of the mainstem bronchus in children were treated with cryotherapy. The narrowing was successfully relieved in one child, whereas cryotherapy was unsuccessful in relieving the obstruction in the other.

Lastly, we have treated three patients for airway tumors with endotracheal cryotherapy. One patient had successful treatment of a subglottic hemangioma with two applications of cryotherapy. The second patient had successful eradication of a neuroblastoma of the arytenoid cartilage with two applications of cryotherapy, and the third patient had successful cryotherapy ablation of a tumor in the subglottic airway of minor salivary gland origin.

CONCLUSION

In our experience, cryotherapy has been successful in relieving obstructing lesions of the airway in 30 of 33 surviving patients (91%). Only three of the children who have been referred to us in the last 11 years will require more extensive open procedures for relief of their obstructions.

The technique of cryotherapy has the advantage of requiring relatively simple and inexpensive equipment. In addition, experimental studies have indicated that the trachea is resistant to extreme degrees of cryotherapy, and there seems to be a wide margin of safety with this technique.[11,17] There have been no major complications as a result of the therapy in our patients, and there has been no instance of airway perforation with this equipment.

Our success in treating neoplasms of the airway with cryotherapy suggests that this may be an important application of the modality in the future. A more efficient coolant, however, must be used in the treatment of large neoplasms. A liquid nitrogen cryoprobe capable of reaching temperatures of $-190°C$ is now available for endoscopic use, and experimental studies utilizing this probe indicate the safety of its application in the airway. The potential for cryoimmunization may provide still additional benefit in the treatment of patients with airway neoplasms.

REFERENCES

1. Adzick NS, et al: Cryotherapy of subglottic hemangioma. J Pediatr Surg 19:353–357, 1984
2. Bracco D: Historical developments. *In* Ablin RJ (ed): Handbook of Cryosurgery. New York, Marcel Dekker, 1980, pp 15–68
3. Carachon R, et al: The place of cryosurgery in the treatment of subglottic angiomas of the infant. Clin Otolaryngol 2:207–211, 1977
4. Carpenter RJ, Neel HB, Sanderson DR: Cryosurgery of bronchopulmonary structures. Chest 72:279–284, 1977
5. Cooper IS, Lee SA: Cryothalamectomy-hypothermic congelation: A technical advance in basal ganglia surgery. Preliminary report. J Am Geriatr Soc 9:714–718, 1961
6. Fraser JD: History and development of cryosurgery. *In* Holden HP (ed): Practical Cryosurgery. Chicago, Year Book Medical Publishers, 1975, pp 1–9
7. Gorenstein A, Neel HB, Sanderson DR: Transbronchoscopic cryosurgery of respiratory structures. Experimental and clinical studies. Ann Otol Rhinol Laryngol 85:670–678, 1976
8. Holden HB, Saunders S: Cryosurgery: Its scientific basis and clinical application. Practitioner 210:543–550, 1973
9. Jokinen K, Palva A, Karja J: Cryocauterization in the treatment of subglottic hemangioma in infants. Laryngoscopy 91:78–82, 1980
10. Le Pivert PJ: Basic considerations of the cryolesion. *In* Ablin RJ (ed): Handbook of Cryosurgery. New York, Marcel Dekker, 1980, pp 15–68
11. Neel HB, et al: Cryosurgery of respiratory structures. I. Cryonecrosis of trachea and bronchus. Laryngoscope 83:1062–1070, 1973
12. Pusey WA: The use of carbon dioxide snow in the treatment of nevi and other lesions of the skin. JAMA 49:1354–1356, 1907
13. Rodgers BM, Rosenfeld M, Talbert JL: Endobronchial cryotherapy in the treatment of tracheal strictures. J Pediatr Surg 12:443–449, 1977
14. Rodgers BM, Talbert JL: Clinical application of endotracheal cryotherapy. J Pediatr Surg 13:662–668, 1978
15. Sanderson DR, Neel HB, Fontana RS: Bronchoscopic cryotherapy. Ann Otol Rhinol Laryngol 90:354–358, 1981
16. Sheperd J, Dawber RPR: The historical and scientific basis of cryosurgery. Clin Exp Dermatol 7:321–328, 1982
17. Thomford NR, et al: Morphologic changes in canine trachea after freezing. Cryobiology 7:19–26, 1970
18. Whittaker DK: Mechanisms of tissue destruction following cryosurgery. Ann R Coll Surg Engl 66:313–318, 1984
19. Zacarian SA, Stone D, Clater M: Effects of temperatures on microcirculation in the golden hamster cheek pouch. Cryobiology 7:27–39, 1970

chapter 11

Endoscopic Electrosurgical Resection of Subglottic Stenosis

Dale G. Johnson, M.D.

Electrosurgical resection through a rigid endoscope is a convenient and useful method of treating selected cases of upper airway obstruction. The technique has been useful for excision of chronic scar, granulation tissue, and benign tumor in the upper airway and is presented here as one among several current therapeutic choices for the management of difficult airway problems in children.

Not all cases of upper airway obstruction are suitable for electrosurgical resection; in properly selected patients, however, it can be the method of choice. The technique, with the aid of some experience, is simple, the equipment is readily available in most pediatric surgical units, and the brief hospitalizations required for resection, although multiple, are usually cost effective. As with most therapeutic modalities, however, the details of proper technical application are closely tied to the degree of success achieved. A poorly executed procedure can cause far more harm than good; the factors I believe are important for a successful endoscopic electrosurgical resection are, therefore, the subject of this chapter.

PATIENT SELECTION

The primary advantage of electrosurgical resection is simplicity for both surgeon and patient. Disadvantages associated with the modality include limited application for complex lesions, the potential for worsening of stenosis by improper application, and a success rate that is highly dependent upon the skill and experience of the surgeon. It should be noted that the latter two disadvantages are shared by all approaches. If the tracheal stenosis in question involves mature, hypertrophic, rigid scar tissue over 5 to 10 mm in thickness or if there appears to be instability of the upper airway secondary to destruction of cartilage, some of the more complicated treatment methods described in this book would probably be preferable to electrosurgical resection. For properly selected lesions, however, endoscopic resection of an upper airway obstruction with short bursts of a low-wattage, pure cutting current is effective, efficient, and inexpensive.

DEVELOPMENT OF THE PROBLEM

Acquired subglottic stenosis in infants following endotracheal intubation is a relatively new problem. The condition appeared approximately 25 years ago in conjunction with the development of long-term intubation techniques and systems for ventilatory support.

Mechanical trauma to the subglottic trachea is associated with tightly fitting endotracheal tubes, poor fixation of tubes, and transmitted motion from a cycling ventilator. The duration of intubation, the size of the infant, and the presence or absence of associated infection are important factors as well. Mucosal injury actually occurs at the point where the endotracheal tube fits most tightly within the trachea, namely, the rigid cricoid ring where the child's trachea is narrowest.

Subglottic stenosis appears to have occurred much more frequently in the early years of its diagnosis than is the case now. Reports between 1965 and 1976 recorded an incidence of 1.7% in 61 cases,[1] 1.6% in 126 cases,[6] 4.7% in 656 cases,[3] and 6.7% in the 263 intubated infants seen during 1976 in our own neonatal intensive care unit.[5] Now, more than 10 years later, the prevailing practice of avoiding tightly fitting endotracheal tubes has produced a gratifying reduction in our own incidence of subglottic stenoses; other facilities report that they have experienced the same result. Current protocols include acceptance of a small air leak, better stabilization of tubes, control of infection, and minimization of intubation times. Some units, working with these protocols, claim to have achieved an idealistic goal—the virtual disappearance of any experience with subglottic stenosis.

The problem, however, will never completely disappear. We see, in addition to the mostly preventable cases of postintubation subglottic and tracheal stenosis, the occasional congenital, neoplastic, postinfectious, and post-traumatic stenoses. Post-tracheostomy granulomas and airway deformities must also be managed; when severe, they require the same type of approach to operative treatment.

CLINICAL EXPERIENCE

In the past 14 years, we have had 55 patients who required surgical treatment for obstructive lesions of the upper airway. Seven of the lesions were thought to be congenital, 3 post-traumatic, 5 postinflammatory, 36 as a result of endotracheal intubation, and 6 of unknown origin or due to other causes. Electrosurgical resection using an infant-sized or specially modified child-sized urethral resectoscope was performed as either partial or full treatment in 38 of the patients. Electrosurgical resection alone was successful in 30 patients. Four of the failures withstood additional procedures by other surgeons involving open

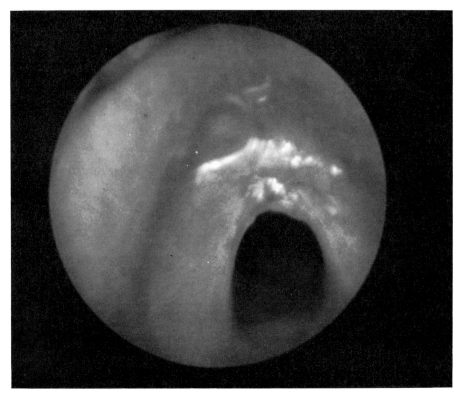

FIGURE 11-1. Horseshoe-shaped diaphragm of subglottic scar successfully treated by electrosurgical resection in three stages.

reconstruction and/or laser resection. We performed open laryngotracheoplasties on the four remaining patients after achieving poor results with electrosurgical resection.

Eight patients were treated successfully with one electroresection only. Seventeen required two resections, seven had three resections, three had four resections, two had five resections, and one had six resections. Eight patients, each of whom had only one or two resections each, were successfully treated without the need for prior tracheostomy. All of the patients with five or six resections and one of the three patients with four resections required subsequent open laryngotracheoplasties before they were successfully decannulated. Our success rate with electrosurgical resection alone, therefore, was 79%.

Thirty-nine of our total 55 patients with tracheal obstructive lesions required a tracheostomy during treatment; the same was true in 30 of the 38 cases managed by electrosurgical resection. The fact that eight symptomatic obstructions were resected successfully without the protection of a tracheostomy suggests that electrosurgical resection may be useful in the management of moderately difficult lesions. Photographs of a few representative lesions treated successfully by the technique alone are presented in Figures 11–1 through 11–3.

It is tempting to think that a physician's accumulated experience may now allow him or her to select the more complicated cases of tracheal obstruction for early laryngotracheoplasty. In so doing, the success rate with electrosurgical resection would be improved and the cost and frequency of open reconstruction cases would be lessened. Whether a surgeon can select cases for laryngotracheoplasty with accuracy, however, remains to be seen. Some patients with near total occlusion of the airway have experienced dramatic success with elec-

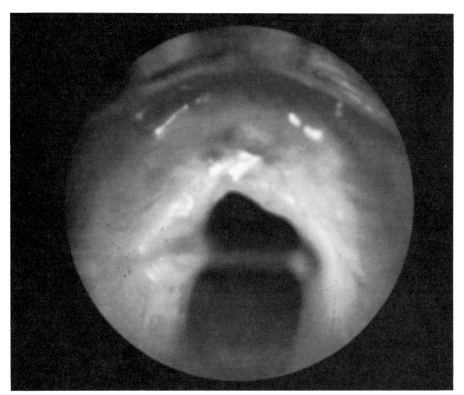

FIGURE 11-2. A 4-mm stenosis divided by a transverse band of scar. Electrosurgical resection of the transverse band was followed by two additional anterior and lateral resections. The resultant airway remained open with no recurrence of stenosis.

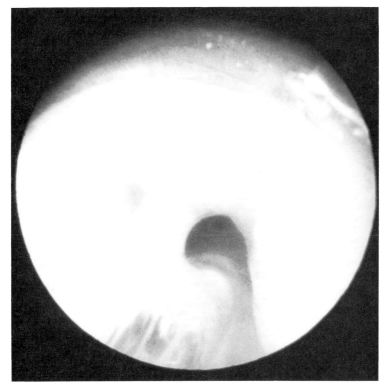

FIGURE 11-3. A thick, tightly scarred, 3-mm subglottic stenosis successfully managed with five resection sessions. The initial view appears discouraging and offers no indication for success. The first electrosurgical resection nevertheless produced dramatic improvement. Subsequent resections resulted in a 6-mm lumen at the cricoid level, which was maintained long term.

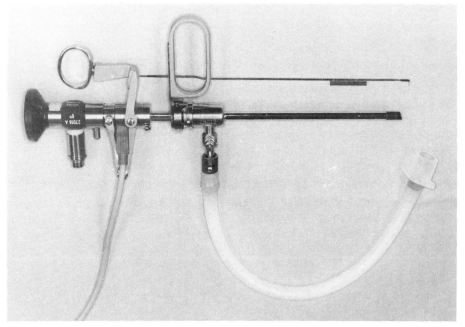

FIGURE 11-4. The infant urethral resectoscope with cutting loops, working mechanism, and sheath. A longer sheath with appropriate loops is available for use with older children.

trosurgical resection; others, cases apparently not so severe, have gone on to require more complicated treatment.

EQUIPMENT

Resectoscopes

The infant urethral resectoscope (K. Stortz*) was the only applicable instrument available when we first reported our technique of electrosurgical resection in 1975.[2] With minor modifications, however, this equipment serves us well. Other manufacturers undoubtably offer a similar instrument, but we remain satisfied with our initial choice. The resectoscope is pictured in Figure 11-4.

The infant scope, with a sheath of 20 cm in length, is adequate for the majority of cases of subglottic stenosis in infants; larger children require a 30-cm scope. Our resectoscope was initially custom made for us by Stortz; it is now, however, commercially available.

Cutting Loops

A variety of straight and ovoid cutting loops have been useful for us in electrosurgical resection of tracheal lesions. On three patients, we used only the cold knife attachment, which can be applied with the manipulative precision and telescopic control of the resectoscope. The cold knife also provides a safe and easy solution for the treatment of webs or bridges of scar beneath the cords

*Stortz Endoscopy-America, Inc., Los Angeles, CA.

requiring only simple incision. With the development of laser technology, however, laser ablation may provide an even better option than resection with a cold knife, but only if the lesion can be aligned precisely with the laser micromanipulator.

Radiofrequency Current Generator

The equipment for generation of the radiofrequency cutting current used in endoscopic resection must be capable of producing an energy output ample enough to cut the subglottic scar but sufficiently restrictive to minimize heat diffusion and thermal damage to adjacent tissues. Many of the standard electrosurgical current generators in operating rooms are too imprecise for the demands of this technique. The proper generator for endoscopic resection is equipped with adjustment controls scaled from 1 to 100 instead of the usual 0 to 5.

Precise limitation of the energy delivered from the cutting current generator is an important factor in the minimization of damage to surrounding tissue; it is also a factor often overlooked when surgeons unfamiliar with endoscopic resection attempt the technique. Some inexperienced physicians have referred to electrosurgical resection as "cautery excision"; this incorrect reference is precisely the type of error that must be avoided. Application of the "cautery" or coagulating current to the tracheal wall is an excellent way to produce experimental subglottic stenosis. In an important study in lambs, we created subglottic stenosis of an impressive and significant degree with the coagulating "cautery" current and then resected the stenoses successfully with the radiofrequency cutting current.[4] The difference between "coagulating" and "cutting" current is the key to success with this technique.

Closed Circuit Ventilation

Control of the airway is simple when a tracheostomy is in place; it is for this reason that tracheostomy prior to resection of subglottic stenosis is a necessity in all severe or complicated cases. Eight of our cases, however, had either one or two successful resections without the inconvenience of prior tracheostomy.

Endoscopic resection without distal tracheostomy requires specialized equipment and technique. The water irrigation ports on the urethral resectoscope should connect with the sheath of the resectoscope, which is inside the trachea. Adapter tubing can then be used to make a closed circuit connection between the resectoscope sheath and the anesthesia machine via the irrigation connector (Fig. 11–5). This arrangement provides a small channel of fairly high resistance; the patient, however, can be monitored with a pulse oximeter. Satisfactory oxygen saturation can be maintained in this manner during a resection if the procedure is done expeditiously.

If oxygen saturation should drop, it is a simple matter to withdraw the loop and manipulator from the sheath, which can then be capped with a glass window. The size of the airway within the sheath is thereby greatly increased, and the anesthesiologist is given satisfactory control of ventilation.

As a precautionary measure, although the danger of intratracheal ignition of gases is small with the use of nonexplosive and nonflammable anesthetic

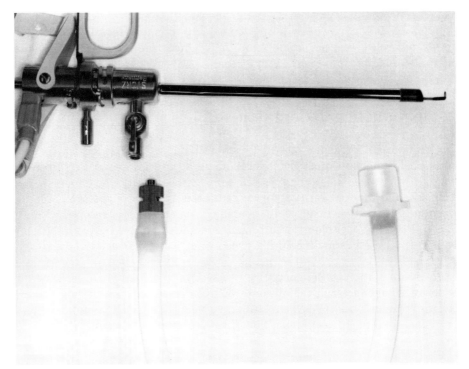

FIGURE 11-5. To maintain ventilation during a resection, the anesthesia machine is connected to the irrigating channel of the resectoscope. The connecting tubing and adapters are shown here. Owing to the small diameter of the channel and the high resistance, the operator must work quickly and efficiently while the patient is monitored continuously with a pulse oximeter.

agents, we stabilize the patient on room air without increased oxygen concentration before beginning the brief period of electrosurgical resection.

Suction Catheters

Fine-bore suction catheters, in small and large sizes and rigid enough to be guided easily and passed in and out of the open resectoscope sheath, should be available during endoscopic resection. The small catheters can often be passed alongside the sheath to withdraw smoke and fumes during resection. The larger catheters are used for the removal of blood and tissue fragments through the lumen of the resectoscope sheath.

TECHNICAL PROCEDURE

Sterile Technique

Endoscopic resection is an intratracheal operative procedure and should be performed with both sterile equipment and sterile technique. Diagnostic procedures in the airway are often performed with clean (as opposed to sterile) scopes and techniques; this concession is not acceptable, however, when the mucosal barrier is invaded by resection. We drape the patient's head and chest and arrange the instruments on a sterile instrument table. Gloves and gowns are worn by both nurse and surgeon.

Preparation and Testing of Equipment

The diagnostic bronchoscope and the resectoscope should both be prepared and tested before insertion into the airway for endoscopic resection. It is helpful to dip the distal end of the telescopes in an antifog or soap solution (Septisol works well) to avoid clouding of the view when the scope is inserted into the warm environment of the trachea. The ventilating tubing should be connected to the irrigation channel, the cutting loop should be connected to the electrosurgical current generator, and any *coagulating current should be turned off*. As discussed earlier, the coagulating current creates stenoses; we aim to resect them.

Endoscopic Evaluation

Inspection of the obstructing lesion is first accomplished with the rigid telescopic bronchoscope, the smallest sheath for which has an external diameter of 4 mm. The lumenal diameter associated with most significant subglottic stenoses in infants is smaller than 4 mm; therefore, it is usually necessary to remove the outer sheath and pass only the 2.7-mm diameter telescope through the stenosis to estimate its thickness. Even the 2.7-mm scope, however, will not always pass through the stenosis. Estimates of thickness can then be made somewhat inaccurately by passage of a small suction catheter through the constricted area. When the stenosis is this severe, prior tracheostomy is always required; as such, owing to the presence of the tracheostomy, airway compromise is seldom a concern during the initial endoscopic evaluation.

For endoscopic evaluation, the patient should be placed in the "sniffing" position with the neck partially flexed forward and the head extended on the neck (Fig. 11–6). To discern and evaluate anatomic details of the supraglottic, glottic, and subglottic airways, the bronchoscope should always be passed through the airway under direct vision through the telescope.

Lesions ideal for resection appear fairly mature and resemble a discrete diaphragm with a thickness of less than 2 mm. The surrounding mucosa does not look boggy, edematous, or inflamed, and the stenosis appears localized and discrete. Lesions of this description favor an easy, successful resection; unfortunately, however, they are the ideal and, as such, are infrequently seen. We have been successful, on three occasions, with much less desirable circumstances, namely, an occlusion through which a 1-mm catheter could not be passed and a stenotic area that appeared to be thick, shaggy, and actively inflamed. Given the situation, it was necessary to cut a channel through the center of the stenosis with the resectoscope to evaluate the thickness of the lesion.

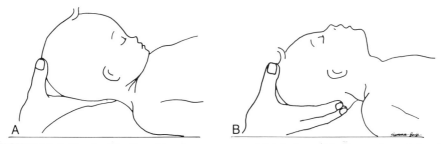

FIGURE 11–6. The "sniffing" position for exposure and intubation of the larynx in an infant is achieved by (*A*) flexion of the neck on the chest and (*B*) extension of the head on the neck.

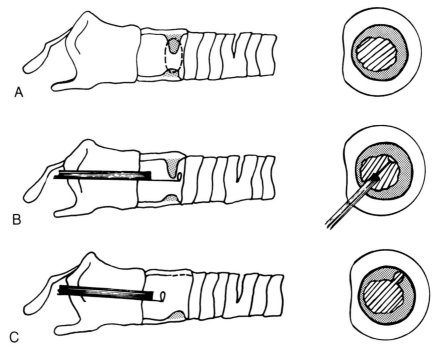

FIGURE 11-7. *A,* Electrosurgical resection is initiated by inserting the resectoscope through the vocal cords under direct vision and positioning the telescope just proximal to the stenosis. *B,* The cutting loop is then extended through the stenotic lumen and placed immediately behind the rim of the scar. *C,* Short bursts of low-wattage, radiofrequency cutting current are then applied to the scar as the loop is withdrawn toward the telescope and insulated sheath.

We consider single-quadrant trial resection to be worthwhile in nearly every case owing to the fact that a successful result is often achieved from a condition that, at first evaluation, appears to be very discouraging. We try to avoid denudation of tracheal cartilage with deep excision, but, on occasion, we have cut through the cricoid anteriorly to expand the cricoid ring.

Resection Technique for Subglottic Stenosis

Endoscopic resection of a subglottic lesion is performed by extending the cutting loop through the stenotic lumen (if there is one) and then pulling the loop, which functions as a hook, against the far side of the stenotic wall (Figs. 11–7 through 11–9). *Short, intermittent bursts of low-wattage cutting current* are applied as the loop is drawn toward the operator and into the insulated portion of the resectoscope sheath. The short pulses of current needed to provide precise control during excision can be produced by quick taps on the foot pedal. The current is initiated at a low setting and adjusted upward until a cutting effect is obtained. The final current setting will vary according to the generator; on a scale of 1 to 100, we use a setting of 10 to 15 (SSE4 Electrosurgical Current Generator*), which we then adjust with widely spaced, intermittent taps on the foot pedal to avoid heat build-up in the tissue touching the loop. *The avoidance of heat diffusion to surrounding tissue is the most important technical detail of endo-*

---

*ValleyLab, Boulder, CO.

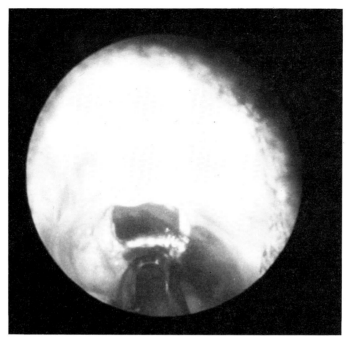

FIGURE 11-8. A semicircular cutting loop positioned behind the anterior rim of subglottic scar in a child with subglottic stenosis.

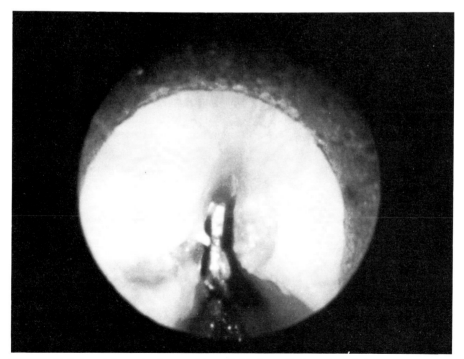

FIGURE 11-9. A straight cutting loop positioned behind a wall of anterior subglottic scar in a child's trachea. The channel in front of the loop was cut by the first pass of the loop through the scar.

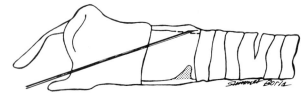

FIGURE 11–10. Intralesional steroid injection following resection of subglottic scar. In practice, the injection needle is passed through the instrument channel of the infant telescopic bronchoscope; in effect, positioning of the needle tip can be controlled by observation through the telescope.

scopic excision. Excess wattage, continuous application of electrical energy, incorrect use of coagulating current, excessive cutting, and too extensive resecting at one sitting can all lead to a greater degree of scarring than is necessary and guarantee a poor result.

A circumferential subglottic scar is usually resected in quadrants; in effect, the posterior midline and the risk of entering the esophagus are both avoided. Esophageal injury, of course, is unlikely if the stenosis is located at the cricoid ring. The precise level of the lesion, however, is not always clear, and the three-quadrant excision is usually sufficient.

Steroid Injection

Following endoscopic resection, it has been our practice to inject a mixture of triamcinolone (40 mg/ml) and hyaluronidase (150 μ/ml) in 0.1-ml increments, mixed 5 ml/1 ml, into the resection site (Fig. 11–10). It has been our hope that steroid injections might soften residual scar and lessen the chance of scar reformation; unfortunately, we have only anecdotal impressions regarding the effectiveness of this practice.

Resection of Other Intratracheal Obstructions

Other lesions, such as polypoid granuloma at the tracheostomy site, subglottic hemangioma, and postintubation granuloma lower in the trachea, are easily removed with the resectoscope; resection, in fact, is nearly always accomplished in a single procedure. The technical aspects of the resection are the same as those discussed for subglottic stenosis. To ensure that it has no contact with the tracheal wall, the cutting loop is always placed distal to the lesion in the trachea. The loop is then brought toward the operator, connecting with and cutting through the lesion as it is withdrawn into the insulated sheath. This procedure provides complete visual control for the operator and eliminates any chance that the loop will cut through an unexpected structure. Note that the application of cutting current while the loop is being extruded distally is unsafe; the object cut in this manner is beyond, rather than between, the loop and the optical telescope and therefore out of the operator's range of vision.

Postoperative Management

Providing the patient has had a protecting tracheostomy before surgery, most cases of endoscopic resection can be managed in an outpatient surgery unit.

Without antibiotic suppression, the raw intratracheal surface becomes colonized and produces thick, purulent secretions; with this knowledge, the postresection child is commonly sent home on antibiotic coverage (usually amoxicillin) for 5 to 7 days. A second evaluation or resection is scheduled for 2 to 4 weeks following the initial operation. This time frame allows for resurfacing of the resected area and permits a more accurate evaluation of what was accomplished at the first resection.

Patients with mild stenoses and no protecting tracheostomy may be resected in one or two stages; the area of resection is then injected with triamcinolone, as detailed previously. A loosely fitting endotracheal tube is positioned within the trachea and left in place for 12 to 24 hours after surgery. The tube provides the patient with an ample airway and compresses both postresection and post-injection swelling. These patients must be monitored, at least overnight, in an intensive care unit; we also cover them with antibiotics for 5 days. Systemic dexamethasone (2 mg/5 kg), administered 12 hours before attempted extubation, may also be helpful.

DISCUSSION

No single method for the management of subglottic stenosis is universally applicable or uniformly successful. The most complex stenoses (those involving the complete circumference of the airway and extending over 1 cm in thickness) usually require open reconstruction, with or without interposition grafting and stenting.

Laser resection is a convenient method for the management of lesions that can be exposed sufficiently to meet the line-of-sight requirements of the CO_2 laser. Laser transmission through a flexible fiber solves most of the problems related to difficult access. At the time of this writing, however, there is no available flexible fiber for the CO_2 laser, the instrument that, for its ablative effect, remains the most effective and discrete source of energy. Flexible fibers for laser transmission are available for a variety of other wavelengths, and the proper laser, with a simple and effective fiber-tip manipulator, may become the method of choice for resection in the future. As a note of caution, however, our earlier studies using flexible-fiber transmission of the Argon and Nd:YAG (Neodymium:Yttrium-Aluminum-Garnet) lasers in the resection of experimental subglottic stenosis in sheep demonstrated two things: (1) the red-specific Argon laser was ineffective for cutting white scar and (2) the Nd:YAG, at least at the energy levels we tested, produced excessive heat diffusion and surrounding tissue injury. Electrosurgical resection, when applied as described previously, produced a zone of surrounding thermal injury similar or slightly greater than that of the CO_2 laser.[4]

Open procedures with interposition cartilage grafting have also been used extensively by others and, with success in complicated cases, by our division. These procedures are of much greater magnitude and potential risk than endoscopic resection, and, as such, we prefer to reserve them for back up in complex cases.

Advantages

The outstanding advantage of electrosurgical resection is simplicity. In addition, the equipment is inexpensive and the resection can be accomplished fairly quickly and expeditiously. Although multiple procedures are usually required, they are generally done on an outpatient basis. None of the alternative procedures can promise a one-stage cure, and most are more complex and expensive than electrosurgical resection. Under telescopic control, the resectoscope loop can be positioned with accuracy at any point within the trachea. Although, owing to its precise nature, the CO_2 laser is clearly superior for the resection of lesions located at or above the cord level, the resectoscope offers a useful and easily applied alternative for those strictures at various levels below the cords.

Disadvantages

Disadvantages of electrosurgical resection were discussed earlier. Suffice it to say, the possibility always exists—in all methods of treatment—for a poor result. Excessive current, the wrong type of current, and steady application of current can each pose significant problems. Adjacent tissue can burn with resultant slough, contraction, and reformation of scar possibly worse than before treatment. In an effort to avoid this situation, a single trial resection is appropriate and should be performed for most lesions. When the result is unsuccessful or the initial lesion is thick and rigid and there is significant deformity of the cartilaginous wall, electroresection should be abandoned in favor of another method.

SUMMARY

Successful management of upper airway obstructing lesions requires flexibility and a variety of therapeutic approaches, each dependent upon the location, severity, maturity, and cause of the obstruction. Endoscopic electrosurgical resection offers a simple and inexpensive first-line approach to treatment; timing and careful restriction of applied thermal energy, however, are critical to the modality's success.

In our hands, electrosurgical resection followed by steroid injection was successful in relieving stenosis and allowing tracheal decannulation in 30 of 38 cases treated by this method alone. The treatment interval varied from 2 to 35 months, with an average span of 9 months. An additional 18 cases were selected for other methods of treatment after initial endoscopic evaluation. These treatments ranged from simple dilatation with steroid injection to laser resection, cricoid and tracheal incision with interposition graft, and segmental sleeve resection of the stenotic trachea with end-to-end anastomosis.

We continue to believe that endoscopic electrosurgical resection has a place in the therapeutic armamentarium for upper airway obstructions. The application of this technique is highly dependent upon the experience, skill, and preference of the surgeon. The modality has proven to be useful in our hands for most, but certainly not all, cases of upper airway obstruction.

REFERENCES

1. Allen TH, Steven IM: Prolonged endotracheal intubation in infants and children. Br J Anaesth 37:566–573, 1965
2. Johnson DG, Stewart DR: Management of acquired tracheal obstructions in infancy. J Pediatr Surg 10:709–717, 1975

3. Lindholm CE: Prolonged endotracheal intubation. Acta Anaesthesiol Scand (Suppl) 31:1–131, 1969
4. Mayer T, Matlak ME, Dixon J, et al: Experimental subglottic stenosis: Histopathologic and bronchoscopic comparison of electrosurgical, cryosurgical, and laser resection. J Pediatr Surg 15:944–952, 1980
5. Parkin JL, Stevens MH, Jung AL: Acquired and congenital subglottic stenosis in the infant. Ann Otol Rhinol Laryngol 85:573–581, 1976
6. Rees GJ, Owen-Thomas JB: A technique of pulmonary ventilation with a nasotracheal tube. Br J Anaesth 38:901–906, 1966

part 4

General
Techniques

chapter 12

Anesthesia for the Child with Airway Problems

Norman H. Brahen, M.D.
Joanne M. Conroy, M.D.
Charles T. Wallace, M.D.

Anesthesia for surgery on the pediatric airway demands expertise in anesthetic planning and management. The first priority is to maintain satisfactory gas exchange via a clear airway. Some degree of airway compromise is usually present (foreign body, edema, or stenosis). In addition, when the airway is shared, such as during bronchoscopy or tracheoplasty, there is a greater potential for complications. Teamwork, close cooperation, and an understanding of both the surgical and anesthetic procedures are essential. Communication between the surgeon and the anesthesiologist must begin during the preoperative planning and continue into the operation as the need for minor adjustments and modifications arises.

PREOPERATIVE EVALUATION

The preoperative assessment of a patient with airway obstruction is imperative for the delineation of possible problems as well as for the formulation of a safe plan of action. A questionnaire completed by the patient or parents preoperatively can considerably facilitate the preanesthetic assessment.[19] A history relating to onset, duration, and nature of symptoms should be elicited. Congenital causes such as choanal atresia, laryngomalacia, subglottic stenosis, congenital webs, and craniofacial abnormalities should be sought. Common acquired causes for airway obstruction should be identified (e.g., laryngotracheobronchitis, foreign body aspiration, and epiglottitis). In addition to the patient's medical history, a history of previous anesthetic experiences, medications, and allergies should be noted.

The physical examination should focus on the airway and the respiratory and cardiovascular systems. The examination should include observations of the color of the mucous membranes; presence of mouth breathing; respiratory rate; condition of teeth; size of tongue; and evidence of respiratory distress (stridor, nasal flaring, retractions, tracheal tug, and anxiety). Mandibular size and the ability to open the mouth and extend the neck will be important in alignment of the various anatomic axes necessary for visualization of the glottis. Patency of the nostrils is tested simply by alternate occlusion. Signs of right-sided heart failure secondary to chronic airway obstruction should be elicited. Palpation and auscultation of the neck and chest may reveal the level of obstruction and establish baseline information necessary for interpretation of intraoperative changes. Indirect laryngoscopy provides valuable information about the site, extent, consistency, and vascularity of obstructive lesions and the mobility of the vocal cords. Roentgenograms of the chest and neck should be studied. Computed tomography (CT) of the neck may further delineate laryngeal and tracheal deviation and compression. Pulmonary function tests, flow volume studies, and arterial blood gas studies are helpful in selected patients.

PREMEDICATION

Premedication should be individualized. Administration of sedatives and narcotics may result in loss of normal muscle tone and cause airway obstruction and depressed ventilatory drive. Thus, they should not be given to patients with airway dysfunction. Anticholinergic agents such as atropine and scopolamine decrease the volume of oral secretions. In addition, both are vagolytic and may be protective against bradycardia, which occurs during endotracheal intubation, surgical stimulation, or hypoxemia. Atropine, because of its superior vagolytic effects on the heart and lack of sedation, should be given intravenously at the time of induction in a dose of 0.02 mg/kg. Preoperative cimetidine reduces gastric acidity and may be helpful in children with full stomachs or gastroesophageal reflux.[8] Because the child will be unsedated, it is of great importance to spend as much time as possible with the child to develop a trusting relationship.

INDUCTION

The techniques used for induction of anesthesia will differ according to the amount of airway disease and the degree of respiratory distress. No matter which technique is used, it is helpful to develop an alternate approach should the initial intubation attempt fail. In our practice, we have categorized patients into four basic groups that dictate the way we manage the induction and intubation.

Type I Patients

These patients have mild airway distress, normal respiratory rate, minimal stridor, a normal blood oxygen saturation, and an outwardly normal upper airway and exhibit mild or nonexistent sternal retractions.

Type II Patients

These patients may have serious respiratory disease and may be in moderate distress but have a "proven airway" (i.e., these children have undergone the procedure previously or a laser procedure, endoscopic tracheoplasty, or bronchoscopy). The anesthesia and surgical teams are familiar with the airway and know which approaches to intubation are successful.

Type I or II patients generally receive an inhalational induction with halothane and oxygen while monitors are applied. When they have passed through the second stage of anesthesia, intravenous access is established. With a good mask fit, 5 to 10 cm H_2O end-expiratory pressure is applied to the airway. This maneuver helps to overcome soft tissue obstruction. Assisted ventilation should gradually be increased to confirm one's ability to ventilate the patient. At this point, atropine (0.02 mg/kg) and succinylcholine (2 mg/kg) are given intravenously and the patients are intubated.

Type III Patients

These patients may or may not be in any degree of respiratory distress. However, their airway anatomy is obserevd to be abnormal, i.e., micrognathia, macroglossia, severe palatofacial deformity, or large tumors that encroach on the upper airway. This group also includes children with lower airway lesions or large anterior mediastinal masses that would be difficult to manage once a general anesthetic and neuromuscular blocking agents are administered.

Type IV Patients

These patients present for the first time with significant airway obstruction. They exhibit obvious respiratory distress with rapid respiratory rate, sternal retractions, low blood oxygen saturation (cyanosis), and obvious signs of fatigue.

The children of both Type III and Type IV require special preparation in anticipation of a difficult direct laryngoscopy and intubation. Equipment and personnel for immediate establishment of an airway must be available, including a needle catheter for cricothyroidotomy and a surgeon experienced in performing pediatric bronchoscopy and tracheostomy.

Older children in this group may tolerate airway manipulation and intubation in the awake but sedated state. Incremental doses of midazolam (0.05 to 0.1 mg/kg) or diazepam (0.1 to 0.2 mg/kg) may be given intravenously for sedation. The nasal passage is then sprayed with a vasoconstrictor (e.g., Neo-Synephrine) and a local anesthetic (2% lidocaine). After the posterior pharynx has been anesthetized, the larynx is anesthetized using 4% lidocaine transtracheally. A nasotracheal tube is then passed into the posterior pharynx and either advanced blindly or with the use of a flexible bronchoscope into the trachea.[7,17] In an uncooperative child or infant, an inhalational induction with halothane can be applied in increasing concentrations until a deep level of anesthesia is achieved. Intravenous lidocaine (1.5 mg/kg) may be effective in depressing airway reflexes if given 1 minute before laryngoscopy. Laryngoscopy should not be attempted until the masseter muscles are completely relaxed and the systemic arterial pressure decreases at least 20% of control values. There are two reasons for maintaining spontaneous ventilation while intubating the patient. First, should neuromuscular blockade be administered, total airway obstruction can occur because the muscle tone of the tongue and cervical and laryngeal muscles is lost. This obstruction may not be relieved by manual ventilation. Second, if the patient is not breathing, a valuable guide to locating the glottis is lost (i.e., bubbles on expiration). With the patient under deep inhalational anesthesia, breathing spontaneously, the posterior pharynx is anesthetized and an "oxyscope" laryngoscope,* which has a sideport for supplemental oxygen, is gently inserted. If tracheal intubation is not completed in 90 seconds anesthesia must be resumed to prevent a return to light levels of anesthesia and accompanying laryngospasm. After repositioning the patient and trying another laryngoscope blade, alternate techniques may be required including blind nasal intubation,[2] use of an anterior commissure laryngoscope,[9] use of a Bullard laryngoscope,† retrograde passage of a guide wire through the cricothyroid membrane,[3] and blind oral intubation using a lighted stylet containing the Flexi-Leum surgical light.[1,5] In the case of anterior mediastinal tumors, the size and location of the tumor and the amount of cardiovascular compromise may necessitate prompt institution of partial cardiopulmonary bypass using the femoral vessels.[13]

AIRWAY ENDOSCOPY

Bronchoscopy

The most common indications for bronchoscopy include evaluation of hoarseness or stridor, removal of vocal cord polyps, foreign body retrievals, tracheobronchial toilet, and examination prior to decannulation.

Bronchoscopy is performed after the patient has received muscle relaxation and has been intubated with a smaller than normal endotracheal tube. The table is turned 15 to 30 degrees before surgical manipulation of the airway and bronchoscope placement. Most commonly, a Storz bronchoscope‡ with a 15-mm adapter for direct connection to the anesthetic circuit is used. Anesthesia is maintained with inhalational agents and 100% oxygen. Frequently, small doses of narcotic are used to supplement the anesthetic. Ventilation is impaired with the telescope in place. Depending on the size of the bronchoscope, the diameter may be decreased as much as 70%.[20] Adequate ventilation can be accomplished by using higher ventilatory pressures and 100% oxygen. Realistically, the pressure transmitted to the tracheobronchial tree is only a fraction of the pressure measured proximally. Ventilating through this diminished cross-sectional area can cause air trapping, barotrauma, and compromised cardiac output. These problems can be alleviated by periodic removal of the telescope with improvement in the ability to ventilate. The anesthesiologist can take advantage of periods of frequent suctioning to occlude the proximal end of the bronchoscope and return to normal ventilation. Using these techniques, the arterial PaO_2 and $PaCO_2$ will remain within acceptable ranges.

---

*Foregger Co., Inc., Smithtown, NY.

†Circon ACMI, Stamford, CT.

‡Karl Storz, Endoscopy American, Inc., Culver City, CA.

Intraoperative cardiac arrhythmias are most commonly associated with hypoventilation and hypoxia. They may be treated by placing the bronchoscope above the carina and increasing ventilation with oxygen. Bronchospasm may also occur and may be treated by increasing the depth of anesthesia.

The potential for anesthetic pollution of the operating room environment is of concern. Attempts are made to stop ventilation except when the telescope, or "window," is in place. At the completion of the procedure the airway is reintubated by the anesthesiologist using a tube at least one size smaller than usual. The patient is allowed to regain airway reflexes and demonstrate adequate neuromuscular functioning before extubation. Postextubation stridor is treated with humidified oxygen or racemic epinephrine (for body weight <10 kg, 0.25 ml of 2% racemic epinephrine in 2 ml normal saline; >10 kg, 0.50 ml of 2% racemic epinephrine in 2 ml normal saline) as necessary. If acute deterioration occurs during or after the procedure, a pneumothorax should be ruled out.

SURGICAL PROCEDURES

Endoscopic Tracheoplasties

During tracheal dilation procedures, a balloon catheter is placed and left inflated at 40 to 80 cm H_2O, depending on balloon size, for 1 to 2 minutes. The management of these cases differs slightly from that of bronchoscopy in that the anesthesiologist must prepare for periodic apnea, 2 to 3 minutes in duration, while the balloon is inflated and deflated. However, after adequate preoxygenation and ventilation with an inhalation anesthetic, we have seen very few problems with desaturation or CO_2 retention during these brief periods.

Laser Excision

Initially, the patient is induced and the airway secured with a small unlubricated endotracheal tube. Lubrication is avoided because of the well-documented combustibility of oil-based lubricants. Special care is given to eye and skin protection. Once the suspension laryngoscope is placed by the surgeon, a Sanders injector is placed in the groove of the scope and the endotracheal tube is removed. Ventilation is continued with oxygen and nitrous oxide in an attempt to maintain an oxygen concentration at less than 40% to minimize the risk of airway fire.[4,15] Muscle relaxation is continuously assessed with a peripheral nerve stimulator since the consequences of a misdirected beam can be devastating and ventilation may become difficult because of laryngospasm. Prior to starting the laser excision, excursion of the chest, auscultation, and noninvasive oxygen saturation assessment are carried out so that small changes can be made in the position of the suspension laryngoscope as necessary. Because potent inhalation anesthetic agents cannot be used, anesthesia is maintained with combinations of IV narcotics, barbiturates, benzodiazepines, and ketamine. Attention is given to titration of muscle relaxants and anesthetics so that the patient has return of airway reflexes and gains consciousness shortly after the conclusion of the procedure. Occasionally, an aluminum-wrapped red rubber tube with a saline-inflated cuff or a Silicon-coated tube is used.[14] Most children, however, can be managed with supraglottic ventilation, allowing greater surgical exposure. Occasionally, we ventilate with a subglottic catheter when jetting through the laryngoscope is inadequate. More commonly, a subglottiscope is used with a short jet catheter. The major complications of either technique are air trapping and barotrauma. Of concern to many is the pounds per square inch (PSI) delivered by the reducing valve present on all these ventilators and blenders. The PSI required for adequate ventilation varies tremendously with the type of scope, the ventilator needle, the length and shape of the needle, and the position of the jet ventilator in the airway.[11] As with all of these ventilation systems, every breath must be examined by observing the chest excursion and auscultating breath sounds.

Foreign Body Retrieval

One of the few airway problems in which an endotracheal tube is not routinely placed prior to bronchoscope insertion is the retrieval of a foreign body. In doing so we hope to avoid dislodgement and possible complete obstruction of the airway. Spontaneous ventilation is maintained, and the scope is inserted under a deep inhalational technique after topical anesthesia of the larynx is performed. Additional lidocaine can be sprayed through the suction port of the bronchoscope. Depending on the nature of the foreign object, patients may or may not need intensive respiratory therapy and racemic epinephrine postoperatively.

Tracheal Resection

Aggressive airway management of the pediatric airway and respiratory care have increased the incidence of acquired tracheal stenosis in infants and children. Treatment for acquired stenosis includes repeated dilation, insertion of a stent, and resection with end-to-end anastomosis when the stenosis lies in the middle or lower part of the trachea. Congenital tracheal stenosis, although uncommon, is usually more extensive and may occur at any level of the trachea.[18] Anesthesia for dilation and stent insertion may be carried out as discussed previously. The anesthetic management for surgical resection is dictated by the location of the lesion.

Glottic or subglottic lesions almost always require tracheostomy for airway access. Following inhalation induction through the tracheostomy site, an armored endotracheal tube can be inserted through the tracheostomy under sterile conditions and sutured into place. At the termination of operation, the tube is replaced by a tracheostomy tube.

Midtracheal lesions can be managed by a small endotracheal tube placed translaryngeally past the site of the lesion.[10] The induction should be by inhalational anesthetic or ketamine to allow the patient to ventilate spontaneously until intubated. The complete relaxation that occurs with neuromuscular blocking agents may produce complete obstruction of the airway. Therefore, they should be avoided until the endotracheal tube is in place and nonobstructed ventilation is initiated. It may be impossible to pass the tube beyond the lesion, and therefore rigid bronchoscopy must be available. Frequent blood gas and acid-base determinations necessitate an indwelling left radial arterial catheter. A left radial artery line should be used because the innominate artery, which crosses the trachea, may be compressed during operation. As the procedure progresses, a second sterile armored endotracheal tube may placed by the surgeon and passed distal to the lesion after the trachea is open. After the posterior anas-

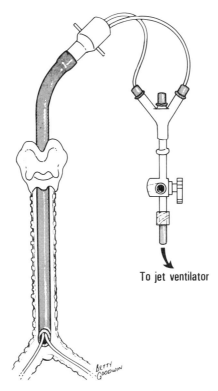

FIGURE 12-1. Diagram of apparatus for ventilation of patients with low tracheal lesions.

tomosis is completed, the second tube is removed and the original tube is advanced distal to the anterior anastomosis.

A number of approaches to the maintenance of anesthesia during operation for distal trachea repair in the pediatric patient have been reported. They include retrograde tracheal intubation with intermittent positive pressure ventilation,[12] passing of a small catheter down the lumen of the endotracheal tube into the distal trachea using high-frequency jet ventilation,[5] and placement of a tracheal T tube with occlusion of the extraterminal limb with intermittent positive pressure ventilation.[16]

We have used two thin polyethylene catheters placed endobronchially under direct vision in a sterile fashion. They are attached to a high-frequency jet ventilator as shown in Figure 12–1. With this technique, ventilation is accomplished by exposing the lungs to rapid intermittent high fresh gas flow from the catheters. Acceptable blood gas levels have been maintained, and there have been no deleterious effects on circulation. With only small catheters in the field, the surgeon can more easily perform the tracheal resection and anastomosis.

Postoperatively, patients are kept in a position of head flexion to reduce tension on the suture line. Early extubation is highly desirable to minimize the compromise of blood flow to the trachea, which might be caused by a snug tube.

REFERENCES

1. Berci G, Katz R: Optical stylet: An aid to intubation and teaching. Ann Otol 88:828–831, 1979
2. Berry FA: The use of a stylet in blind nasotracheal intubation. Anesthesiology 61:469, 1984
3. Borland LM, Swan DM, Lett S: Difficult pediatric endotracheal intubation: A new approach to retrograde technique. Anesthesiology 55:577–578, 1981

4. Burgess GE, Lejeune FE Jr: Endotracheal tube ignition during laser surgery of the larynx. Otolaryngology 105:561–562, 1979
5. Ellis DG, Jakymec A, Kaplan RM, et al: Guided orotracheal intubation in the operating room using a ligated stylet: A comparison with direct laryngoscopic technique. Anesthesiology 64:823–826, 1986
6. Ellis RH, Hind CJ, Gadd LT: Management of anesthesia during tracheal resection. Anesthesia 31:1076–1080, 1976
7. Fan LL, FLynn JW: Laryngoscopy in neonate and infants: Experience with flexible fiberoptic bronchoscope. Laryngoscope 91:451–456, 1981
8. Goudsouzian N, Cote CJ, Liu LMP: The dose-response effects of oral cimetidine on gastric pH and volume in children. Anesthesiology 55:533, 1981
9. Handler SD, Keon TP: Difficult laryngoscopy/intubation: The child with mandibular hypoplasia. Ann Otol Rhinol Laryngol 92:401–404, 1983
10. Lee P, English ICW: Management of anesthesia during tracheal resection. Anaesthesia 29:305–306, 1974
11. Miyasaka K, Sloan IA, Froese AB: An evaluation of the jet injector (Sanders) technique for bronchoscopy in paediatric patients. Canad Anaesth Soc J 27:117–124, 1980
12. Nelrand M, Tseudo K, Browning S: Anesthesia for extensive resection of congenital tracheal stenosis in an infant. Anesth Analg 58:431–433, 1979
13. Northrip DR, Bohman BK, Tseuda K: Total airway occlusion and superior vena cava syndrome in a child with an anterior mediastinal tumor. Anesth Analg 65:1079–1082, 1986
14. Ossoff RH, Eisenman TS, Duncavage JA, Karland MS: Comparison of tracheal damage from laser-ignited endotracheal tube fires. Ann Otol Rhinol Laryngol 92:333–336, 1983
15. Pashayan AG, Gravenstein JS: Helium retards endotracheal tube fires from carbon dioxide lasers. Anesthesiology 62:274–277, 1985
16. Rah KH, Griffith RL, Jones JJ: Anesthetic management of the pediatric patient with a tracheal T-tube. Anesth Analg 60:445–447, 1981
17. Rogers SN, Benumot JL: New and easy techniques for fiberoptic endoscopy-aided tracheal intubation. Anesthesiology 59:569–572, 1983
18. Samaan HA: Benign tracheal stenosis. Br J Surg 57:909–913, 1970
19. Steward DJ: Anaesthesia for paediatric outpatients. Canad Anaesth Soc J 27:412–416, 1980
20. Woods AM, Gal TJ: Decreasing airflow resistance during infant and pediatric bronchoscopy. Anesth Analg 66:457–459, 1987

chapter 13

Pediatric Endoscopy

Stephen L. Gans, M.D.

Direct examination of the larynx provides a true image of its anatomy and pathology and is the initial step in the examination of the tracheobronchial tree. Bronchoscopy is quite indispensable in the study of endotracheal and endobronchial conditions, for it provides information for diagnosis and a method of treatment unobtainable in any other way.

It is important to understand normality and its variations to appreciate both common pathologic conditions and rarities. Although it is understood that practical instruction and clinical experience cannot be replaced, instruments presently available allow close observation of both laryngoscopy and bronchoscopy by means of teaching attachments and video transmission. These devices also facilitate documentation and video recording for both clinical use and detailed study. The bottom line, however, is that mastery of manipulative techniques through the bronchoscope is achieved only through practice.

Environment and Personnel

Laryngoscopy and bronchoscopy are most effectively and safely performed in an operating room or a specially designed and equipped endoscopy room. Advantages to this sort of setting include adequate space, sterile technique, resuscitative ability, and the availability of a full range of facilities, which optimally includes x-ray and ultrasound equipment.

Well-trained personnel should include an anesthesiologist, an experienced head holder, a scrub nurse trained in endoscopic technique, and a circulating nurse. It is also helpful and instructive for an endoscopic assistant or trainee to be present. In addition, particularly in the case of a neonate or sick child, a neonatologist or pediatrician is an important member of the team. Such nonsurgical physicians can profit from the opportunity to visualize directly certain pathologic conditions they are called upon to treat.

Anesthesia

Given the presently available anesthetics and endoscopes and pediatric anesthesiologists experienced in endoscopic technique, general anesthesia is the method of choice for endoscopy. Full sedation permits the performance of an unhurried, safe, thorough, and complete procedure with a minimum of physical and psychological trauma to the patient and surgeon alike.

LARYNGOSCOPY

In older children, the larynx and pharynx can often be inspected by indirect examination under light sedation and with a laryngeal mirror. This procedure, however, is not feasible in infants, and direct examination under general anesthesia is almost always indicated. In addition to providing adequate ventilation, anesthesia provides relaxation of the mandible and pharynx to permit gentle and leisurely examination, depression of the vagal reflex, and, in many cases, retention of vocal cord movement to allow assessment of the dynamics of the pharynx and larynx. Occasionally, in sick neonates or those with suspected vocal cord paralysis, no anesthetic is used; however, the presence of an anesthesiologist is advisable.

Preparation

Except in an emergency situation, appropriate radiologic studies, scans, or ultrasound should be performed before anesthesia is initiated (Fig. 13–1). The use of premedication and anesthetic techniques will vary according to the experience and preference of the anesthesiologist.

Equipment

Many useful laryngoscopes are available with proximal and distal bulb lights or fiberoptic light sources. My preference is the Storz pediatric laryngoscope,* which is available in several sizes. Of note is a special-model laryngoscope that has a spoon-shaped blade designed to keep the tongue from slipping off to the side and a built-in channel through which a suction tube can be passed; with this type of scope, the physician is able to accomplish simultaneous aspiration and examination without the need to switch hands.[2]

Detailed inspection can be carried out with either the short, rigid telelaryngoscope (Storz) or the telescopic bronchoscope, particularly if continuation into tracheobronchoscopy is planned. For endolaryngeal microsurgery, a self-retaining, self-supporting laryngoscope and microlaryngeal instruments with an attached microscope are available (Fig. 13–2). These instruments permit accurate diagnosis and precise laryngeal manipulation, including the use of lasers, cautery, and cryotherapy.[1]

---

*Storz Endoscopy America, Los Angeles, CA.

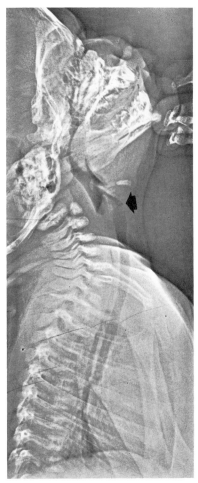

FIGURE 13–1. A lateral xerogram of a normal infant showing the upper airway from the bronchi below through the trachea, larynx, pharynx, nasopharynx, and nasal airways. The arrow indicates the laryngeal ventricle. (Reprinted with permission from Benjamin B: Laryngoscopy. *In* Gans SL (ed): Pediatric Endoscopy. New York, Grune & Stratton, 1983.)

Photodocumentation, cinematography, and video recording devices are available for attachment to those telescopes with suitable light sources. Sensitive, light-weight video cameras permit a clear, magnified view on a monitor during recording (Fig. 13–3).

Method

The patient is placed in the supine position on a regular, horizontal operating table. A general anesthetic is administered through a face mask. The examination is begun when the anesthesia reaches the required depth. After a topical anesthetic is applied, the laryngoscope is introduced while the child breathes spontaneously. With the tongue lifted, the scope is passed behind the epiglottis; the endolarynx is then exposed by raising the laryngoscope with the left hand. Care is taken to retract the upper and lower lips to protect them from trauma

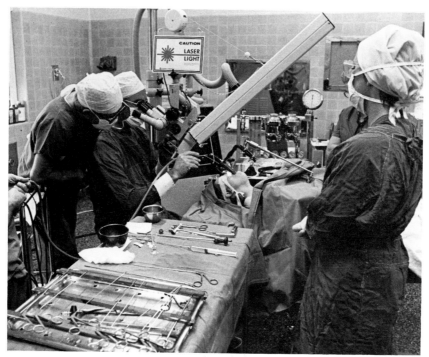

FIGURE 13–2. The self-retaining laryngoscope rests on a support over the patient's chest, and the surgeon has both hands free for operative micromanipulation, in this case with a laser. (Reprinted with permission from Benjamin B: Laryngoscopy. *In* Gans SL (ed): Pediatric Endoscopy. New York, Grune & Stratton, 1983.)

and avoid injury to the teeth. The head and neck are adjusted appropriately to facilitate exposure, while the operator's right index finger is placed on the anterior neck to manipulate the larynx as needed (Fig. 13–4).

Examination focuses primarily on the larynx. When indicated, however, examination is extended to include the oropharynx, the base of the tongue and valleculae, the pyriform fossae, the postcricoid region, the epiglottis, the arytenoids, the false cords, the ventricles, the vocal cords, the subglottic region, and the upper trachea. If more detailed examination is indicated, anesthesia is appropriately deepened and the laryngoscope is reintroduced. In such instances, short, rigid telescopes, such as the Hopkins rod lens by Storz, with straightforward or angled views, give a clear, wide-angle, magnified image with which to evaluate the anatomic structures (Fig. 13–5). These telescopes are also useful for photographic or video tape documentation (see Fig. 13–3).

BRONCHOSCOPY

When pediatric bronchoscopy is performed, adequate safety, sufficient time for careful intubation, and complete examination and treatment of the bronchial tree are of prime importance. Present-day anesthesia and modern instruments have enabled physicians to meet these priorities in most circumstances. Preparation of a child for bronchoscopy is similar to that previously described for laryngoscopy.

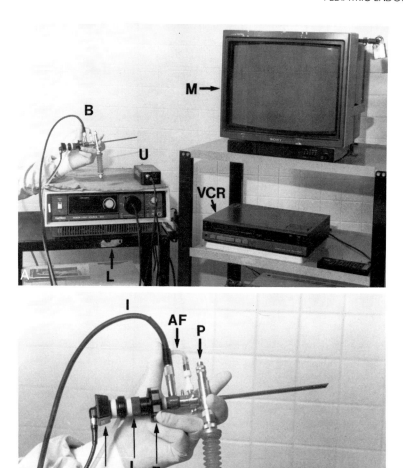

FIGURE 13–3. *A*, Bronchoscope (*B*) provided with miniature video camera connected to camera control unit (*U*) and, thereby, to video camera recorder (*VCR*) and monitor (*M*) for viewing. Xenon light source (*L*) provides illumination through fluid light cable. *B*, Close-up miniature bronchoscope with illumination provided by light cable (*I*), antifog sheath *(AF)*, prism light (*P*) for proximal illumination when telescope is removed, and ventilator or anesthesia connector (*V*). The miniature video camera (*C*) and lens (*L*) are clipped onto the eyepiece (*E*) and connected to the camera control unit (*U*).

Equipment

The development of miniature telescopes and their use in conjunction with fiberoptic lighting have increased the safety and accuracy of bronchoscopy.[3] The superior view not only provides a sharp, magnified, wide-angle image, making orientation easy and quick, but also affords sufficient light for photodocumentation, video recording, and split-image teaching attachments. In addiion, there is enough space remaining in the bronchoscope sheath in miniature telescopes for both adequate ventilation and/or anesthesia and a number of

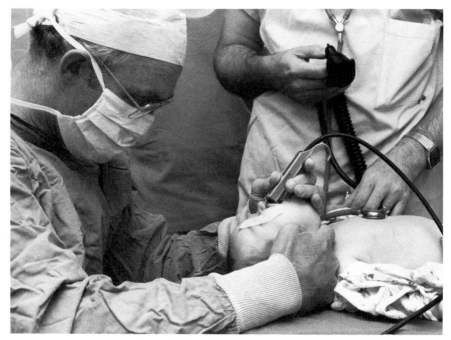

FIGURE 13-4. Direct laryngoscopy with the child breathing spontaneously. Note the index finger on the child's neck to manipulate the laryngeal structures for ready visualization. (Reprinted with permission from Benjamin B: Laryngoscopy. *In* Gans SL (ed): Pediatric Endoscopy. New York, Grune & Stratton, 1983.)

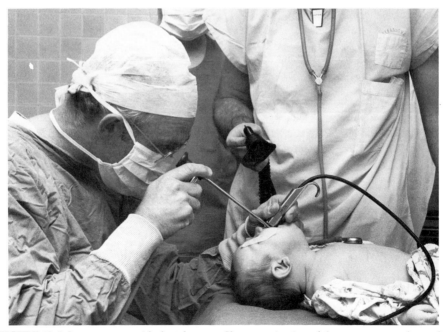

FIGURE 13-5. Laryngoscopy with the telescope. Close examination of the structures can be made with bright illumination, a clear image, and minimal trauma. (Reprinted with permission from Benjamin B: Laryngoscopy. *In* Gans SL (ed): Pediatric Endoscopy. New York, Grune & Stratton, 1983.)

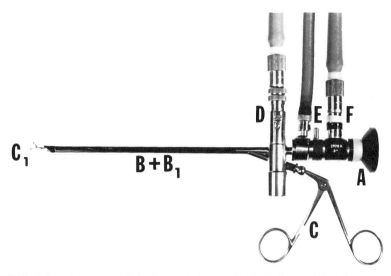

FIGURE 13–6. Bronchoscope with foreign body forceps blades in front of the telescope end. Eyepiece of the telescope (*A*), which extends through the entire bronchoscope, with distal light provided by fiberoptic connection (*F*) through fibers associated with the telescope. Proximal light source (*D*) provides light through the empty bronchoscope sheath by means of a prism. The bronchoscope sheath (*B* + *B₁*) includes an inside antifog sheath through which air is blown from an air pump connected at *E*. A foreign body forceps handle (*C*) has the forceps in position in the instrument channel and operating tip of the forceps (*C₁*) in front of the telescope. (Reprinted with permission from Gans SL: Bronchoscopy. *In* Gans SL (ed): Pediatric Endoscopy. New York, Grune & Stratton, 1983, p 53).

manipulating instruments. Flexible fiberscopes now provide better quality images than their earlier models but have neither the ventilative nor the manipulative instrumentation capabilities of the rigid telescopes, which will be described later.

When treating neonates and infants, we use the Storz miniature rigid bronchoscopes. All 20 cm in length, the bronchoscopes vary, however, in sheath size from 2.5 to 3.0 to 3.5, these numbers indicating the inside diameter or lumen of the tube. Each is equipped with a Hopkins rod-lens telescope with fiberoptic distal lighting and a proximal prism lighting system (Fig.13–6A and D). The two larger sizes are also provided with "antifog" sheaths through which air is blown by an air pump to keep the lens of the telescope clean (Fig. 13–6B and B₁). Telescopes with viewing angles of 0, 30, and 70 degrees are also available.

A small instrument guide channel is attached obliquely to the sheath for introduction of suction catheters, biopsy forceps, grasping forceps, and electrocautery, all manipulations being done in direct vision through the telescope (Fig. 13–6C and C₁). It is important to note that sufficient room must be left in the sheath during examination to provide ventilation or controlled respiration for the patient; a wide-bore tube on the sheath can be connected to an anesthetic machine or respirator for this purpose. In the very unusual event of inadequate ventilation, the telescope may be temporarily removed and the bronchoscope converted into a wide, closed system by inserting a "window plug" in the end of the bronchoscope (Fig. 13–7A and B).

For larger infants and children, bronchoscope sheath sizes 3.0, 3.5, 3.7, and 4.0 are available in 26-cm lengths and sheath sizes 3.5, 3.7, 4.0, 5.0, and 6.0 are available in 30-cm lengths. These scopes are similarly equipped with appropriate telescopes, proximal prism lights, and antifog tubes. Their instrument chan-

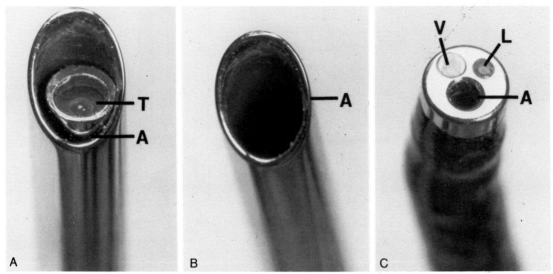

FIGURE 13–7. *A,* End of miniature bronchoscope (size 3.5) with telescope (*T*) and surrounding space for ventilation or anesthesia (A). *B,* Telescope removed, demonstrating wide open airway space. Proximal end of bronchoscope may be closed off with "window plug" (not shown) to provide a closed airway system. *C,* End of same-sized flexible bronchoscope with provisions for light (*L*) and viewing (*V*) and a channel (*A*) for airway, instrumentation, suction, and irrigation.

nels, however, offer a wider variety and selection of manipulating instruments than those previously discussed.

Illumination is provided through fiberoptic cords or cables and produced by a variety of cold-light fountains. The light sources range from small, easily portable units to more complicated and versatile arrangements featuring multiple outlets, variable power, photoflash capabilities, and a xenon light source for photography or video recording.

Advanced-model, flexible pediatric bronchoscopes, such as the Olympus BF-3C10, provide a much better view than did earlier models but have yet to equal the excellent view of the rigid telescopes. Moreover, the flexible bronchoscope fills most of the airway lumen, particularly in the small patient, and provides very little additional ventilatory capability through its suction-instrument channel (Fig. 13–7C). Owing to the small size of the channel, thick secretions are not handled well and instrumentation is quite limited. Foreign body removal, in fact, is contraindicated when flexible scopes are used because they do not allow satisfactory airway control. Flexible bronchoscopes do, however, have limited indications for use in larger infants and children.

A variety of rigid, flexible, and jointed teaching attachments, each with special capabilities, are available for use in older children. Camera adaptors have been developed that fit on the telescope eyepiece or split-image attachment for still and video photography. Late-model miniature video cameras that are fully immersible, such as the Storz Mini Solid State CCD, also clip on; this arrangement allows the physician to perform the procedure while looking through the telescope or at the video screen (see Fig. 13–3).

Technique

The patient is placed on the operating table with the shoulders propped up and a pillow under the head. With a secure intravenous line running and cardiopulmonary monitors in use, the patient's head and body are draped with sterile material. The surgeon, assistant, and endoscopy technician or scrub nurse wear sterile gowns and gloves; all instruments to be inserted in the airway should be sterile.

The prescribed position of the patient during bronchoscopy is flexion of the head and neck on the anterior chest, with subsequent moderate hyperextension of the head on the forwardly flexed neck. This bodily arrangement seems more appropriate for the adult or older child than for younger patients. The neonate and infant are so much more flexible and softer than older children that we have found that *gentleness* in manipulation, with a proficient head holder present, provides all the exposure necessary without unusual postures.[2]

The patient's gums or teeth are protected by a soft, moist sponge, and the laryngoscope is inserted with its tip just at the base of the tongue, pointed toward the suprasternal notch. A lifting motion against the base of the tongue exposes the vocal cords by elevating the epiglottis; at this point, the bronchoscope may be introduced. Note that a common error is insertion of the laryngoscope blade too far, resulting in airway obstruction from laryngeal occlusion and possible trauma to the epiglottis or upper larynx. The tip of the blade should be placed at the base of the tongue (Fig. 13–8A), just proximal to the eipglottis. If forward elevation of the tongue does not, at this point, expose the vocal cords, the laryngoscope blade should be advanced gently, slightly into the vallecula, to elevate the epiglottis and expose the cords (Fig. 13–8B). Again, too deep an insertion will obstruct the airway and hide the cords.

With the glottis exposed by the laryngoscope, the bronchoscope is held like a pencil in the right hand and passed through the cords under direct vision, the physician using the lip of the bronchoscope sheath, if necessary, to separate the cords. The passage into the trachea is then immediately verified (Fig. 13–8C), through the use of the telescope if necessary. Consequently, the telescope is removed, the proximal open end of the sheath is closed with the glass window, and the instrument channel is plugged with a rubber nipple, thereby giving the anesthesiologist a large, closed-circuit airway with which to ventilate and stabilize the patient. When the child's condition has stabilized, the window is removed, the telescope is reinserted, and the tracheobronchial tree is examined. Anesthesia and ventilation are maintained through the large side vent.[2]

An alternative method involves the use of the bronchoscope with the telescope already in place, a functioning suction catheter in the instrument channel, and air blowing through the antifog sheath. With the aid of the bright and detailed view through the telescope, the epiglottis is located and tilted upward with the end of the bronchoscope sheath, which is then passed through the vocal cords in direct view.

Following examination of the trachea (see Fig. 13–8C), the advancing instrument can be directed gently into one bronchus and then into the other by shifting the patient's head from side to side. Photographs or videotapes can then be made as desired. Suctioning may be carried out intermittently or continuously with a fine catheter passed through the instrument channel. This effort actually saves valuable operating time, as it maintains a clear field during inspection. For more extensive suctioning with a larger catheter or tube, the telescope is removed and the suction tube is passed down the main channel of the sheath. In these instances, the distal end of the telescope should be dipped in warm water and wiped free of any foreign matter before reintroduction into the airway.

Fogging of the tip of the telescope lens is effectively prevented by use of anti-

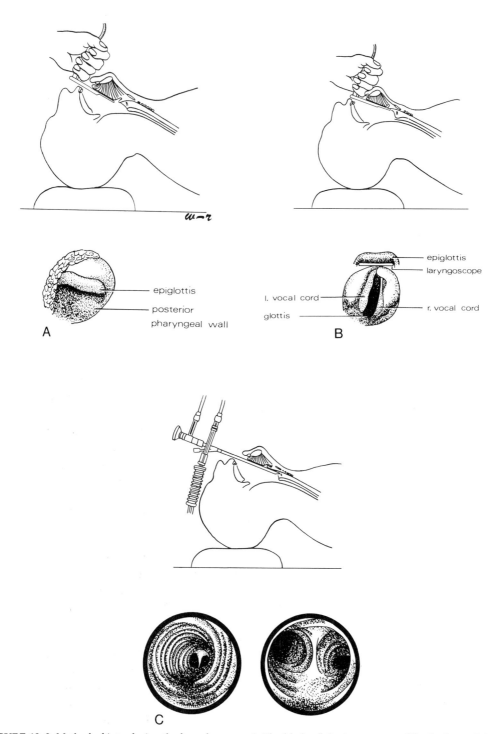

FIGURE 13–8. Method of introducing the bronchoscope. *A*, The blade of the laryngoscope lifts the base of the tongue, exposing the epiglottis. *B*, The epiglottis is gently lifted, exposing the vocal cords. *C*, The bronchoscope is introduced through the vocal cords into the trachea, and inspection is carried out using the telescope. (Reprinted with permission from Gans SL: Bronchoscopy. *In* Gans SL (ed): Endoscopy. New York, Grune & Stratton, 1983, pp 50–52.)

fog sheaths connected to an air blower. Warming the telescope end in water prior to each insertion of the telescope is an additional aid.

Needles for injection, electrocoagulation tips, and biopsy and foreign body forceps are introduced through the instrument channel as needed and are used in direct view of the telescope. The instrument channel also accommodates small catheters for suction, for instillation of solutions, or for passage through a fistula. A Fogarty catheter is useful for the last-mentioned purpose, and its inflatable balloon can be used for temporary occlusion of the fistula, palpation during an operative procedure for fistula correction, or the removal of a foreign body.

Smooth instruments or catheters can also be passed alongside and outside of the sheath and still be used under direct vision of the telescope.

Complications

Many of the potential complications associated with tracheobronchoscopy in infants and children are life-threatening. The forceful passage of a scope too large for the patient's airway, or the traumatic passage of even the proper sized scope, may produce subsequent edema of the epiglottis, cords, or subglottic area with significant airway obstruction. Perforation of the trachea or bronchus with resultant pneumothorax or pneumomediastinum is possible. The introduction of infection through poor technique and contaminated instruments can also have serious consequences. Finally, inadequate control of ventilation or partial mechanical obstruction of the airway during instrumentation can result in cerebral hypoxia and cardiac arrest. The possibility that any of these complications will occur in the hands of an experienced team has been measurably diminished by the development of miniature equipment, which provides excellent visualization and maintains secure control of ventilation.[2]

REFERENCES

1. Benjamin B: Laryngoscopy. *In* Gans SL (ed): Pediatric Endoscopy. New York, Grune & Stratton, 1983, pp 23–24
2. Gans SL: Bronchoscopy. *In* Gans SL (ed): Pediatric Endoscopy. New York, Grune & Stratton, 1983, pp 42, 48–53
3. Gans SL, Berci G: Advances in endoscopy of infants and children. J Pediatr Surg 6:199–234, 1971

chapter 14

Foreign Bodies in the Pediatric Airway

Ann M. Kosloske, M.D.

Obstruction of the airway or esophagus by a foreign body is a common and potentially fatal pediatric accident. In 1984 alone, choking on food or foreign objects accounted for 271 deaths in children under 5 years of age in the United States.[1] According to a detailed study of 15 such deaths, the majority (60%) occurred in children 12 months of age or younger who suffocated when an object larger than a peanut became impacted at the vocal cords or in the trachea.[29] A national survey of 103 food-related asphyxiations in children implicated the hot dog, an item often impacted in the upper airway or upper esophagus, as the single most common agent of death of this type.[11]

Eighty per cent of the children who aspirate foreign objects are under 3 years of age and two thirds are boys.[2,24] Children at this age lack molar teeth with which to finely chew as well as discretion concerning objects appropriate for ingestion. Peanuts and other nuts account for approximately one half of all inhaled objects; they are followed by vegetable fragments, seeds, popcorn, and an array of miscellaneous toys and objects (Table 14–1). Fortunately, the vast majority of foreign objects inhaled are smaller than the child's upper airway and the accidents they cause are not fatal. The treatment of choice in pediatric airway obstruction by a foreign body is bronchoscopic extraction under general anesthesia.

EMERGENCY MANAGEMENT AT THE SCENE

The child who has aspirated a foreign body and is still breathing should be transported immediately to the hospital; no back blows or other maneuvers should be attempted along the way. In the rare instance in which the child is

168

TABLE 14-1. Types of Aspirated Foreign Bodies in Children:
Composite of 481 Children from Three Series,[2,16,24] 1980–1984

Foreign Body	No. Patients	Per Cent
Peanut or other nut	220	45.7
Vegetable/food fragment	78	16.2
Metallic object (pin, screw)*	37	7.7
Plastic object	37	7.7
Seed/husk	24	5.0
Popcorn	22	4.6
Weed	13	2.7
Bone	11	2.3
Stone*	7	1.5
Crayon	6	1.2
Tooth*	4	0.8
Pen/pencil part	4	0.8
Miscellaneous (chalk, cotton, charcoal)	18	3.7
TOTALS	481	100

*Radiopaque foreign bodies.

turning blue and cannot breathe, an adult should quickly look into the back of the child's throat and remove any visible object caught there. Blind finger sweeps in the pharynx, however, should be avoided; the foreign body may easily be pushed further into the airway during such attempts. It should be noted here that mouth-to-mouth resuscitation is ineffective if the upper airway is completely blocked.

To dislodge the aspirated object, the Heimlich maneuver should be performed. The rescuer should stand behind the child, who may be sitting or standing. The rescuer should then wrap his or her arms around the child and give a sharp upward and inward thrust with the fist against the child's abdomen, just above the navel.[25] This routine, which may also be performed with the child supine and the rescuer kneeling beside the child, may be repeated six to ten times until the object is expelled.

Owing to the risk of injury to intra-abdominal organs by subdiaphragmatic abdominal thrusts, the Heimlich maneuver must always be applied very gently in small children. Recognition of the maneuver's inherent risk led to the 1985 recommendations for pediatric basic life support of choking infants under 1 year of age, which endorse a combination of back blows and chest thrusts as initial treatment.[25] The choking infant should be placed face down across the adult's lap and given four brisk blows to the back. He should then be turned over and given four brisk sternal compressions. Some controversy exists regarding the merits of back blows versus the thrusts of the Heimlich maneuver in children; there should be no hesitation, however, in the use of either on a child who is cyanotic with airway obstruction.[7,10,12] Fortunately, because the aspirated object will typically lodge in one or the other mainstem bronchus, these emergency measures are not often necessary. The child may wheeze or experience episodic coughing but is usually able to ventilate well enough to make it to the hospital.

DIAGNOSIS AND INITIAL MANAGEMENT

A brief history and physical examination of the child should be completed in the emergency room. Immediate "crash" bronchoscopy is rarely necessary in children who have aspirated a foreign body. There is usually sufficient time to obtain x-rays and prepare the patient for general anesthesia. In fact, if the child has a full stomach, bronchoscopy should be deferred for a few hours until general anesthesia can be administered safely.

The child may have ceased coughing by the time he or she reaches the hospital. Inhalation and subsequent impaction of a foreign object initially trigger a violent cough reflex, which may be followed by a latent period as the surface sensory receptors of the respiratory tract undergo normal physiologic adaptation.[22] This quiet interval in which the child is devoid of symptoms may give observers the false impression that the impacted object has been coughed out or swallowed; the admitting physician, however, should not be deterred from further investigation.[9] Classic physical findings in cases of foreign body aspiration consist of unilateral decreased breath sounds as a result of decreased aeration of the lung and unilateral rhonchi due to partial occlusion of the bronchus. Wiseman analyzed the diagnostic findings after aspiration in a study of 157 children.[30] The clinical triad of wheezing, coughing, and diminished or absent breath sounds was present in only 39% of his patients, although 75% had one or more of these findings. Those diagnosed early (within 1 day of aspiration) were less likely to exhibit all three symptoms than those patients diagnosed later (31% versus 47%).

A chest x-ray, with views on inspiration and expiration, should be taken following completion of the child's history and physical. Only 10% of all aspirated foreign bodies are radiopaque (see Table 14–1); the x-ray diagnosis is thus based upon changes secondary to unilateral obstruction of an airway. The classic radiographic abnormality is unilateral emphysema with "air trapping" secondary to the ball-valve effect of a high-grade partial occlusion of a bronchus. In these patients, air enters the affected lobe or lung on inspiration (Fig. 14–1A) but subsequently does not escape on expiration (Fig. 14–1B). Other studies that may demonstrate unilateral air trapping are decubitus views of the chest and chest fluoroscopy. In approximately 25% of all cases of foreign body aspiration,

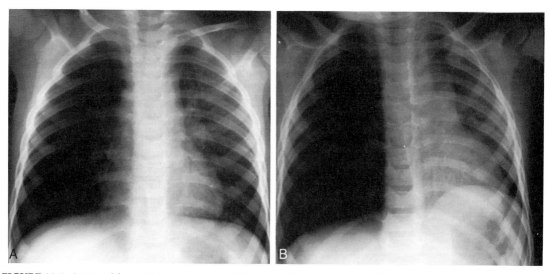

FIGURE 14–1. Aspirated foreign body, right bronchial tree, in a 2-year-old boy. *A,* PA view on inspiration shows emphysema of the right lung. *B,* Emphysema increases markedly on expiration, with mediastinal shift and flattening of the right hemidiaphragm. Six almond fragments were removed from the child's right mainstem bronchus, the bronchus intermedius, and the right lower lobe bronchus by the Fogarty catheter technique.

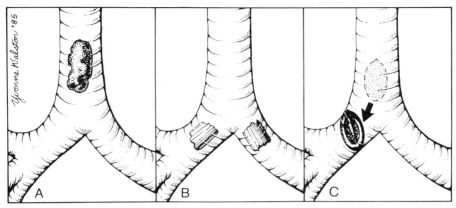

FIGURE 14-2. Normal radiographic findings after foreign body aspiration in children with a tracheal lump of charcoal (*A*), bilateral bronchial crayons (*B*), and a migrating watermelon seed (*C*). (Reprinted with permission from Musemeche CA, Kosloske AM: Normal radiographic findings after foreign body aspiration. When the history counts. Clin Pediatr 25:624–625, 1986.)

total occlusion of a bronchus produces atelectasis or infiltrates rather than emphysema.

It is possible for a child's x-rays and physical examination to be normal in the presence of an aspirated foreign body if the foreign body is lodged in the larynx or trachea (Fig. 14–2*A*) or if bilateral bronchial foreign bodies are present (Fig. 14–2*B*). Furthermore, migration of a foreign body within the airways (Fig. 14–2*C*) may lead to changing physical and radiographic findings. Normal physical findings and normal x-rays do not, therefore, negate the need for bronchoscopy.[20] The child's history of aspiration alone is an indication to proceed.

Approximately 15% of all pediatric aspirations are not observed by an adult. In these instances, the child presents with unexplained wheezing or pneumonia for days or even weeks after the event. Experienced pediatricians and pediatric surgeons can attest to the adage, "all that wheezes is not asthma," particularly as it applies to a 1- or 2-year-old child. Bronchoscopy should always be considered for wheezing of abrupt onset or pneumonia that does not respond to treatment.

A series of treatments involving the inhalation of bronchodilators and chest physiotherapy were advocated by Burrington and Cotton during the 1970s for children who had aspirated foreign bodies.[3] This method, in which the child expels the aspirated object by coughing, proved successful (thereby obviating the need for bronchoscopy) in approximately 25% of patients.[18] The method, however, carried a risk of cardiopulmonary arrest associated with migration of the foreign body within the airways during treatment.[6,17] The authors now limit the inhalation–postural drainage technique to children with small, peripheral foreign bodies and perform bronchoscopy in most cases.[4]

Before a child undergoes bronchoscopy, the parents must be informed of the nature of the procedure, its risks, and any available alternatives. There is a general lack of understanding of the seriousness and potential dangers associated with manipulation of the pediatric airway. Bronchoscopic extraction is a delicate procedure that should be performed by an endoscopist and an anesthesiologist experienced in the care of the pediatric airway. An inexperienced team is more likely to have a difficult extraction or even a major complication during the procedure. As for alternatives, there are no good ones; bronchoscopic extraction is the standard method for removal of a foreign body from the pediatric airway.

TABLE 14–2. Bronchoscopic Equipment for Extraction of a Foreign Body*

Laryngoscope, pediatric
Bronchoscopic tubes, 4.0 mm × 30 cm, 3.5 mm × 30 cm
Slotted antifog sheath for 4.0 mm × 30 cm tube
Telescope (Storz) with Hopkins lens, 0 degrees, 30 cm long
Telescopic bridge adapters (2) for 3.5-mm scope and optical forceps
Optical forceps
Telescope (Storz) with Hopkins lens, 0 degrees, 36.5 cm long, for optical forceps
Light source and cord
Prismatic light deflector
Glass window
Rubber nipples, with and without holes
Suction tubes, metal and plastic
Suction trap
Fogarty catheters, #3 and #4
Forceps, alligator and peanut
Fine foreign body forceps
Dormia stone basket
Magill forceps
Antifog solution
Dilute Neo-Synephrine solution
Sterile aqueous lubricant

*General supplies, such as sterile drapes, warm water, saline, and syringes, and anesthesia equipment are not included on this list.

In preparation for anesthesia, an intravenous cannula should be placed. A dose of penicillin or ampicillin is usually administered, particularly if the child already has pneumonia or the foreign body has been lodged in the airway for more than 24 hours. Finally, atropine should be given before bronchoscopy for foreign body extraction.

INSTRUMENTATION

The state of the art instruments for extraction of foreign bodies are the pediatric bronchoscopes that use the Hopkins rod-lens system.* These instruments are described in detail in Chapter 13. The endoscopist must be both thoroughly familiar with such instruments and capable of assembling and modifying them according to the needs of the extraction. A list of requisite equipment for extraction of a foreign body from the pediatric airway is given in Table 14–2.

The Extraction Procedure

ANESTHESIA AND POSITIONING.   The electrocardiogram (ECG), blood pressure, and oxygenation should be monitored during pediatric bronchoscopy. The pulse oximeter is invaluable during bronchoscopy because it instantaneously records changes in oxygenation and thereby allows the anesthesiologist and endoscopist to adjust the ventilation before any harm occurs from hypoxia. Anesthesia is usually induced by a combination of inhalation agents, oxygen, and intravenous muscle relaxants. The child is supine, i.e., flat on the operating table; the neck is not hyperextended. The child's head is draped and the eyes are taped shut for their protection. Because observation of chest movement aids

*Storz Endoscopy America, Los Angeles, CA.

in evaluation of ventilation throughout the procedure, the child's chest should not be swathed in sheets.

INSERTION OF THE BRONCHOSCOPE. A small laryngoscope with a straight blade is inserted, and the child's vocal cords are exposed. Some endoscopists spray the vocal cords with 1 ml of 1% lidocaine to diminish vagal reflexes during the procedure[21]; others, wishing to retain the child's normal protective reflexes during the emergence from anesthesia, prefer to work with the cords unanesthetized.[5] The pediatric bronchoscope, held like a pencil, with the bevel placed vertically, is then slipped between the cords. Note that the entire bronchoscopic assembly may be inserted into the trachea at once, or, as an alternative method, the outer sheath may be passed into the airway first and the antifog sheath and telescope then slipped into place. The anesthesiologist quickly attaches the ventilation system to the bronchoscope, situated within the trachea, and the procedure begins. Movement of the chest should be observed while the bronchoscope is still in the trachea to confirm the adequacy of ventilation. The trachea is viewed as the scope is advanced toward the carina, and the foreign body is usually visualized in one or the other mainstem bronchus. Once the intruding object has been located, the child's unaffected side is examined briefly to confirm that the area is normal and clear of fragments.

EXTRACTION OF THE FOREIGN BODY. The type and shape of the foreign body determine the optimal instrument for its extraction. We prefer the Fogarty catheter for peanuts and other spherical foreign bodies; seeds, husks, and other flat foreign bodies with an edge are extracted by forceps.

The ideal combination for extraction of a peanut from a mainstem bronchus is the 4-mm Storz bronchoscope, the #4 Fogarty catheter, and 0.4 ml of saline for inflation of the balloon. The bronchoscope is positioned just above the peanut, and any local secretions are suctioned away to provide the endoscopist with a perfect view of the intruding object. A well-lubricated #4 Fogarty catheter is passed down the instrument channel of the bronchoscope and its tip is directed beyond the peanut (Fig. 14–3A). The inner (antifog) sheath of the bronchoscope and the telescope are drawn back approximately 1 cm within the outer sheath; in so doing, a space is created to hold the peanut within the tip of the instrument. The assistant or instrument nurse then inflates the balloon of the Fogarty catheter with 0.3 to 0.4 ml of saline (Figure 14–3B), and the endoscopist gives a gentle pull on the catheter. If the bronchus is small or if the balloon is too tight within it, inflation is decreased until the balloon is able to slide easily within the bronchus. The endoscopist then gently manipulates the catheter until the peanut moves into the tip of the bronchoscope. When this occurs, the anesthesiologist discontinues positive pressure ventilation for a moment as the entire assembly (bronchoscope, catheter, and foreign body) is removed from the airway (Fig. 14–3C). Steady traction is applied to the Fogarty catheter by the endoscopist as he or she watches the peanut during the extraction to ensure that it does not fall back into the airway.

Good communication between the endoscopist and the anesthesiologist is essential for a smooth procedure. As soon as the bronchoscope is removed from the airway, the anesthesiologist should be ready to resume ventilation with a mask. The peanut, however, will occasionally fall back into the child's throat just as the bronchoscope passes the cords. The endoscopist must then quickly insert the laryngoscope and extract the peanut with the Magill forceps. If the peanut is not immediately found, the child should be oxygenated with the mask, after which the operator can examine the pyriform sinuses and posterior pharynx for the intruding nut.

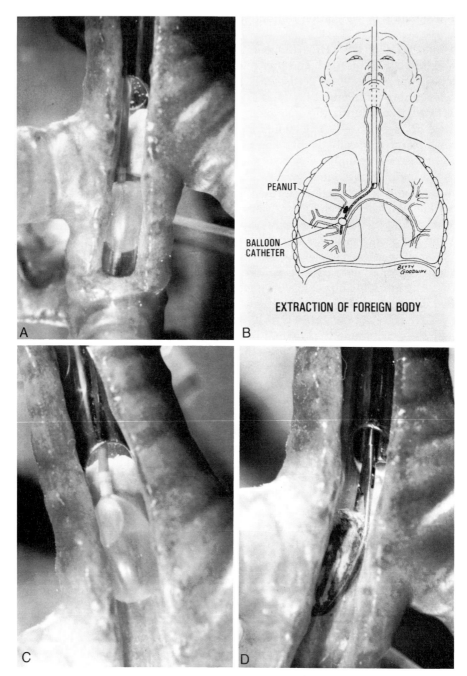

FIGURE 14–3. Methods of extracting various types of foreign bodies are illustrated on a model of the infant tracheobron-chial tree. *A*, Fogarty catheter passed beyond peanut. *B*, Balloon inflated. *C*, Entire assembly (bronchoscope, peanut, and catheter) removed. *D*, Sunflower seed grasped by fine foreign body forceps.

A "second look" at the airway should always be taken to rule out the pres-ence of multiple foreign bodies or retained fragments and to obtain cultures from the affected bronchus. The 3.5-mm bronchoscope, which has an outside diameter of 6.0 mm, provides an adequate view and is less traumatic to the vocal cords than the 4.0-mm scope with its outside diameter of 7.0 mm. The bronchial mucosa at the site where the peanut was impacted is often severely inflamed and may contain a ring of granulation tissue. These granulations will heal once the foreign body has been removed and thus need not be cauterized. Purulent secretions, however, should be suctioned from the distal bronchus and submitted for appropriate cultures. If no additional fragments are present, the bronchoscopic procedure is completed and the scope is withdrawn.

Some endoscopists prefer optical forceps to the Fogarty catheter for the extraction of peanuts.[2,15] Optical forceps, which are designed for foreign body extraction, have a grasping forceps built into the outer sheath of the bronchoscope. Like our preferred method, use of the optical forceps permits extraction of the peanut under magnified direct view.

DIFFICULT PEANUT EXTRACTIONS. Every so often, a peanut that has been in the airways for several days or weeks becomes so tightly impacted that the #4 Fogarty catheter cannot be passed beyond it. The bronchoscope, in such situations, can be rotated through 360 degrees, 90 degrees at a time, in an attempt to pass the catheter on different sides of the peanut. If this maneuver is unsuccessful, a #3 Fogarty catheter with a 0.20-ml capacity balloon may be tried. The optical forceps are yet another excellent alternative, and a third option, one, however, that sacrifices magnification, is passage of the large foreign body forceps into the airway via the central channel. Note that crunching of the softened peanut into multiple fragments in an attempt to suction them away piecemeal is not considered a viable option. Every effort should be made to remove the peanut intact; a second bronchoscopy is preferable to deliberate fragmentation of a peanut. Unable, on one occasion, to extract a mushy, boggy peanut from a mainstem bronchus, we removed the object intact with the Dormia stone basket.

Extraction of a peanut lodged in a child under 1 year of age is a special challenge for the physican because the 4-mm Storz bronchoscope is too large for the patient's small airway. The optical forceps, however, which have an outside diameter of 6.0 mm, may prove suitable. We recently removed a pinon nut from the right mainstem bronchus of a 7-month-old girl using the 3.5-mm Storz bronchoscope and the #3 Fogarty catheter, which does not ordinarily fit down the instrument channel of this size bronchoscope. When both catheter and telescope are well lubricated, however, they can be passed down the 3.5-mm bronchoscope together and moved forward and backward as a unit. This maneuver is not generally recommended because it risks damage to the delicate telescope. In addition, forceful instrumentation of a Fogarty catheter may lead to the complication of separation of the catheter tip within the bronchus.[27] Ingenuity, it seems, is the bottom line for successful extraction of difficult foreign bodies.

EXTRACTION OF FOREIGN BODIES OTHER THAN PEANUTS. Seeds and all other flat foreign bodies are extracted under magnified view using either the optical forceps or the fine foreign body forceps passed via the instrument channel (Fig. 14–3D). When the latter combination is used, the foreign object may be drawn into the tip of the bronchoscope by moving its inner sheath and telescope back 1 cm within the outer sheath; as described earlier, a small hollow is thereby created in the tip of the bronchoscope. Some attention should be paid to the orientation of the flat foreign body; the operator should bring the object vertically, rather than horizontally, through the cords to avoid stripping it from the forceps. The third option for extraction of flat foreign bodies involves the passage of standard forceps via the central channel of the bronchoscope. Because this alternative sacrifices magnification, the bronchoscope should be positioned to allow precise application of the forceps before the telescope is removed.

Stones, screws, and large, sharp foreign bodies present specific problems during removal. Such objects may be too large to grasp with forceps of any type, and those with sharp points may puncture the Fogarty catheter balloon. We have successfully used the Dormia basket, in both the animal laboratory and two children, when confronted with difficult or awkward foreign bodies. Note that a brief practice session with the basket before bronchoscopy is very helpful.

CRISIS MANAGEMENT

THE PATIENT CANNOT BE VENTILATED DURING THE EXTRACTION. This situation may occur when the tip of the bronchoscope is in one of the mainstem bronchi. The bronchoscope should be drawn back into the trachea and the antifog sheath and telescope removed. The anesthesiologist can then easily ventilate the patient with minimal resistance. Lockhart and Elliot documented the high resistance found in Storz bronchoscopic instruments[19]; mechanical difficulties caused by this resistance, however, pose little problem as they can be corrected immediately by simple adjustment of the system.

THE FOREIGN BODY FALLS BACK INTO THE AIRWAY DURING EXTRACTION AND THE PATIENT CANNOT BE VENTILATED WITH THE MASK. The foreign object is probably lodged at the vocal cords or subglottic area if this situation, which constitutes a desperate emergency, occurs. The laryngoscope should be quickly inserted, and, if the object is at the cords, it should be removed with the Magill forceps. If the object is not at the cords, the bronchoscope should be reinserted and, under direct vision, the object either extracted immediately or pushed back into one of the two mainstem bronchi. The latter maneuver will re-establish one-lung ventilation until a successful extraction can be accomplished.

THE ENDOSCOPIST CANNOT SEE ANYTHING. The endoscopist's view may be obscured by secretions, blood, or fog. Secretions should be suctioned away. A dilute topical solution of Neo-Synephrine or epinephrine is useful for rinsing areas of granulation tissue to temporarily stop bleeding. And fog at the tip of the telescope results from a gradient in the patient's body temperature and that of the telescope. Warming the telescope end in water before insertion into the airway, dipping it into antifog solution, or moving the telescope back 5 to 10 mm within the sheath usually dissipates the fog. A brief application of suction or an air blower to the antifog sheath may also clear the view.

THE FOREIGN BODY IS TOO LARGE TO BE BROUGHT THROUGH THE CORDS. Pen caps, displaced stent tubes, and other rigid objects that are larger than the bronchoscope may be stripped off or cause injury to the vocal cords during extraction. Swensson and colleagues described an effective technique for management of this situation.[26] A tracheostomy is performed over the bronchoscope. The large object is then grasped by bronchoscopic forceps and drawn up the trachea to the level of the stoma. Finally, the object is extracted with a hemostat via the tracheostomy. Removal of the tracheostomy is possible within 48 hours if the airway is normal.

THE FOREIGN BODY IS PERIPHERAL OR CANNOT BE REMOVED. A foreign body that is visible in a segmental bronchus but beyond the reach of the bronchoscope may be dislodged with a #3 Fogarty catheter.[15] It may subsequently be extracted with either the #4 Fogarty catheter, which has a larger

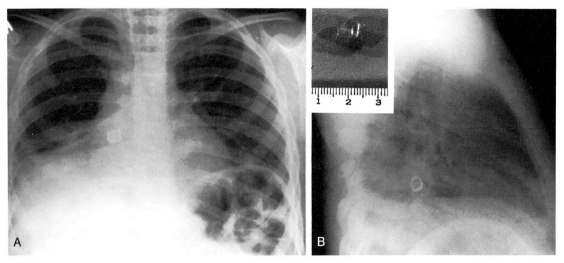

FIGURE 14-4. Peripheral foreign body, a pencil cap, discovered 1 week after aspiration by an 8-year-old Native American boy, with PA (A) and lateral (B) views. An unsuccessful bronchoscopy was performed before referral. Our bronchoscopy was also unsuccessful owing to both granulation tissue, which filled the right lower lobe bronchus, and the peripheral location of the foreign body. The pencil cap (inset) was removed from the medial basal segment of the right lower lobe bronchus with thoracotomy and bronchotomy.

balloon, or the appropriate forceps. Note that bronchography and fluoroscopy may be helpful adjuncts to extraction of a foreign body from a segmental or subsegmental bronchus.[13]

The final consideration for removal of a foreign body that cannot be extracted endoscopically is thoracotomy and bronchotomy, a procedure that we performed only once in more than 100 foreign body extractions. The foreign body in our experience was a pencil cap impacted in a basilar segmental bronchus of an 8-year-old boy (Fig. 14–4). In an effort to diminish the risk of subsequent stricture, linear bronchotomy was performed in the right lower lobe bronchus, just above the take-off of the segmental bronchus. This membranous portion of the bronchus was opened to avoid cutting the cartilage and creating an area of bronchomalacia. The foreign body was then disimpacted by a Penfield elevator passed distally through the bronchotomy and the pencil cap ultimately extracted with forceps. The boy has since had no history of pneumonia or other clinical evidence of bronchial stricture in 7 years of follow up.

NO FOREIGN BODY IS SEEN.   With unilateral physical findings and air trapping on x-ray, infection may occasionally mimic foreign body aspiration. When acute bronchitis is diagnosed at bronchoscopy, washings for culture should be taken and the procedure quickly terminated. If there is a good history of aspiration and no obvious infection, a smaller bronchoscope should be substituted for the one in operation to permit a better look into the lobar and segmental bronchi. Testing for tracheomalacia and bronchomalacia should also be done by allowing the patient to breathe spontaneously under anesthesia and cough while the bronchoscope is positioned within the airway. If the bronchoscopy is negative, esophagoscopy should be considered to rule out the possibility of an impacted esophageal foreign body causing extrinsic compression of the airway. If both bronchoscopy and esophagoscopy are negative for a foreign body, the patient should be followed medically for 2 to 3 weeks. A repeat endoscopy may be considered if symptoms persist.

CHRONIC FOREIGN BODIES

A foreign body retained in the airways for days or weeks is likely to be surrounded by an inflammatory reaction and granulation tissue. Distal bronchiectasis and abscess formation may occur. A chronic retained foreign body usually presents as recurrent pneumonia with, occasionally, a history of hemoptysis. These symptoms are considered a "red flag" and should alert the surgeon to have blood ready at the time of bronchoscopy and bronchography should emergency thoracotomy prove necessary. Massive hemorrhage during extraction of a chronic foreign body has been reported.[23] The classical chronic foreign body is a gross inflorescence (flowering head), which by a rachet effect migrates distally through the small bronchi into the lung substance and even across the pleura.[8,14]

At bronchoscopy, an attempt should be made to localize the segment containing the retained foreign body. This task may be difficult owing to longstanding chronic inflammation and bleeding from granulation tissue; bronchography, however, may prove helpful in localizing the problem. Thoracotomy is necessary for chronic retained foreign bodies that have caused destruction of lung tissue by bronchiectasis.[28] If the damage is localized to a segment rather than to a lobe, consideration should be given to segmentectomy or wedge resection, both of which preserve adjacent normal lung. Lobectomy should be reserved for situations in which multiple segments are destroyed by the inflammatory process.

POSTBRONCHOSCOPY MANAGEMENT

Following bronchoscopy, most children experience some degree of croup from edema of the cords or the subglottic area. The symptoms are apt to be more severe if a large bronchoscope was used in a small patient or if the extraction procedure was lengthy and difficult. We routinely place postbronchoscopy children in a mist tent with 30% oxygen and observe them in either the pediatric intensive care or subacute unit. Also important at this stage in the child's recovery is hydration with intravenous and oral fluids. If obstructive airway symptoms develop, the child should be given inhalation treatments with racemic epinephrine and bronchodilators as needed. Steroids are not routinely given.

Focal bronchitis is common after aspiration of any foreign body. The irritating oils in nuts probably accounted for the surprising 20% incidence of pneumonia we observed in 35 nut aspirations, a percentage significantly higher than the 8% occurrence rate we noted in 38 non-nut aspirations.[18] Antibiotics should be given for bronchitis or pneumonia until clinical evidence of infection has resolved. Chest physiotherapy with postural drainage may also be helpful at this stage for clearing purulent secretions from the affected lobes. If the child's inflammation is severe, parents may be taught to provide chest physiotherapy at home.

A chest x-ray is usually obtained before the postbronchoscopy child is dismissed from the hospital. Residual edema and inflammation may cause persistent x-ray abnormalities. Unless questions remain, however, concerning the adequacy of the first bronchoscopy or if multiple fragments were present in the airway, a repeat bronchoscopy should not be considered until the child has received at least 1 week of treatment with antibiotics and chest physiotherapy at home. Children, like adults, generally recover clinically before their x-rays return to normal. If symptoms or x-ray abnormalities do persist, repeat bronchoscopy for retained fragments should be performed. Bronchography should be considered for longstanding, retained foreign bodies, which predispose to bronchiectasis.

PREVENTION

Foreign body aspirations are, in many instances, preventable accidents. Most parents are unaware of the danger of feeding peanuts and small, particulate foods to young children, a persistent phenomenon that attests to the great need for public education. Warning labels on foods hazardous to young children— peanuts, hot dogs, and popcorn, to name a few—have been proposed and, if accepted, would resemble warning labels on drugs, cigarettes, and dangerous household products.[11] Physicians are currently involved in the diagnosis and treatment of foreign body aspirations; they should next address the root of the problem and contribute to public enlightenment of this significant childhood hazard.

REFERENCES

1. Accident Facts. Chicago, National Safety Council, 1987, p 8
2. Black RE, Choi KJ, Syme WC, et al: Bronchoscopic removal of aspirated foreign bodies in children. Am J Surg 148:778–781, 1984
3. Burrington JD, Cotton EK: Removal of foreign bodies from the tracheobronchial tree. J Pediatr Surg 7:119–122, 1972
4. Campbell DN, Cotton EK, Lilly JR: A dual approach to tracheobronchial foreign bodies in children. Surgery 91:178–182, 1982
5. Cohen SR, Lewis GB Jr, Herbert WI, Geller KA: Foreign bodies in the airway. Five-year retrospective study with special reference to management. Ann Otol Rhinol Laryngol 89:437–442, 1980
6. Cotton EK, Abrams G, Vanhoutte J, Burrington J: Removal of aspirated foreign bodies by inhalation and postural drainage. Clin Pediatr 12:270–276, 1973
7. Day RL, Crelin ES, DuBois AB: Choking: The Heimlich abdominal thrust vs back blows. An approach to measurement of inertial and aerodynamic forces. Pediatrics 70:113–119, 1982
8. Dudgeon DL, Parker FB, Frittelli G, Rabuzzi DD: Bronchiectasis in pediatric patients resulting from aspirated grass inflorescences. Arch Surg 115:979–983, 1980
9. Gans SL: Bronchoscopy. In Gans SL (ed): Pediatric Endoscopy. New York, Grune & Stratton, 1983, p 41
10. Greensher J, Mofenson HC: Emergency treatment of the choking child. Pediatrics 70:110–112, 1982
11. Harris CS, Baker SP, Smith GA, Harris RM: Childhood asphyxiation by food. A national analysis and overview. JAMA 251:2231–2235, 1984
12. Heimlich HJ: First aid for choking children. Back blows and chest thrusts cause complication and death. Pediatrics 70:120–125, 1982
13. Hight DW, Philippart AI, Hertzler JH: The treatment of retained peripheral foreign bodies in the pediatric airway. J Pediatr Surg 16:694–699, 1981
14. Jewett TC Jr, Butsch WL: Trials with treacherous timothy grass. J Thorac Cardiovasc Surg 50:124–126, 1965
15. Johnson DG: Bronchoscopy. In Welch KJ, Randolph JG, Ravitch MM, et al (eds): Pediatric Surgery, 4th ed. Chicago, Year Book Medical Publishers, 1986, pp 619–622
16. Kosloske AM: Bronchoscopic extraction of aspirated foreign bodies in children. Am J Dis Child 136:924–927, 1982
17. Kosloske AM: Tracheobronchial foreign bodies in children. Back to the bronchoscope, and a balloon. Pediatrics 66:321–323, 1980
18. Law D, Kosloske AM: Management of tracheobronchial foreign bodies in children. A re-evaluation of postural drainage and bronchoscopy. Pediatrics 58:362–367, 1976
19. Lockhart CH, Elliot JL: Potential hazards of pediatric rigid bronchoscopy. J Pediatr Surg 19:239–242, 1984
20. Musemeche CA, Kosloske AM: Normal radiographic findings after foreign body aspiration. When the history counts. Clin Pediatr 25:624–625, 1986

21. O'Neill JA Jr, Holcomb GW Jr, Neblett WW: Management of tracheobronchial and esophageal foreign bodies in childhood. J Pediatr Surg 18:475–479, 1983

22. Pyman C: Inhaled foreign bodies in childhood. A review of 230 cases. Med J Aust 1:62–68, 1971

23. Rees JR: Massive hemoptysis associated with foreign body removal. Chest 88:475–476, 1985

24. Rothman BF, Boekman CR: Foreign bodies in the larynx and tracheobronchial tree in children. A review of 225 cases. Ann Otol Rhinol Laryngol 89:434–436, 1980

25. Standards for cardiopulmonary resuscitation (CPR) and emergency cardiac care (ECC). Part IV: Pediatric basic life support. JAMA 255:2954–2960, 1986

26. Swensson EE, Rah KH, Kim MC, et al: Extraction of large tracheal foreign bodies through a tracheostoma under bronchoscopic control. Ann Thorac Surg 39:251–253, 1985

27. Treen DC Jr, Falterman KW, Arensman RM: Complications of the Fogarty catheter technique for removal of endobronchial foreign bodies. J Pediatr Surg 24:613–615, 1989

28. Weissberg D, Schwartz I: Foreign bodies in the tracheobronchial tree. Chest 91:730–733, 1987

29. Weston JT: Airway foreign body fatalities in children. Ann Otol Rhinol Laryngol 74:1144–1148, 1965

30. Wiseman NE: The diagnosis of foreign body aspiration. J Pediatr Surg 19:531–535, 1984

chapter 15

Tracheostomy in Infants and Young Children

J. Alex Haller, Jr., M.D.

The majority of tracheal injuries in infants and children result from iatrogenic or physician-induced causes. Most of these injuries are complications of prolonged endotracheal intubation and difficulties associated with improper performance of tracheostomy. Other causes of chronic tracheal stenosis and upper airway obstruction, such as congenital anomalies and direct external trauma, are extremely rare.

During the 20-year period from 1960 to 1980, the care of neonates developed rapidly. Technological advances soon made possible the resuscitation and ventilation of smaller and smaller premature infants. A large number of these infants had prolonged ventilatory support through endotracheal tubes and subsequently developed subglottic stenosis and other forms of tracheal injury with secondary scarring and obstruction.[7,11] Since 1980, however, the incidence of tracheal injury associated with prolonged intubation, even in tiny, premature babies weighing less than 1000 gm, has decreased remarkably. This improvement is the direct result of several factors: the development of much less irritative materials for the construction of endotracheal tubes,[1] better recognition of the pathophysiology of inflammation and infection associated with indwelling endotracheal tubes, far better protocols for careful inspection of the upper airway, and the frequent changing of tubes by neonatologists with greater experience with tracheostomy.

Although intubation stenoses still occur, most notably in association with major airway infection, they are much less common and rarely result in an indication for operative tracheostomy to ensure the airway. Currently, a major cause of tracheal stenosis requiring subsequent reconstructive procedures and prolonged endotracheal therapy is improperly performed tracheostomy in infants and small children.[8,12,15]

Accepted operative technique for tracheostomy in small infants was critically reviewed in 1974 by Aberdeen and Downes[1] and Haller and Talbert[6]; several causes of post-tracheostomy stenosis and airway obstruction were identified. One of the major etiologies of tracheostomy complication was *emergency operation* in a child without a secured airway. Under circumstances of increasing hypoxemia in an unsedated and squirming child, inadvertent technical mishaps occurred with inexact incision of structures in the neck and rough handling of the underlying trachea. There were often difficulties with intubation once the tracheostomy had been made. Resulting fibrosis from trauma, hemorrhage, and inflammation contributed to the high complication rate.[8,16]

A second major factor found in the incidence of post-tracheostomy stenosis and airway obstruction was the continued use of *metal tracheostomy tubes* with resultant secondary trauma to the surrounding tracheal tissues. As a remedy, soft plastic tracheostomy tubes were introduced by Aberdeen and Downes.[1] These tubes were subsequently refined, and today excellent tubes of soft, silicon rubber or polyvinyl are available with appropriate shapes for the anatomy of the different-sized tracheas in newborns and small infants.[5,6]

The third important observation made by Aberdeen and Downes involved the actual tracheostomy technique. Tracheostomy, they found, was either accomplished by *excising a window of trachea* from the anterior wall or by making a stellate incision, cutting the tracheal rings above and below, and incising laterally to enlarge the opening in the trachea (see Fig. 8–3). Both of these techniques, especially excision of tracheal tissue, resulted in a lack of anterior support of the tracheal wall. Consequently, during attempts to decannulate the trachea, the soft tissues of the neck often fell into the tracheostomy opening, thereby rendering decannulation difficult if not impossible. The presence of inlying, soft tissues also resulted in increased granulation tissue, prolonged healing, and subsequent fibrosis and stenosis at the tracheostomy site.

As a result of these observations and subsequent studies,[9,10,13] a standard operative technique for tracheostomy in infants and young children has evolved. This protocol is based on the physician's understanding of underlying complications that result in stenosis and the importance of preventing injury by delicate handling of the fragile tissues of an infant's trachea.[6,16]

PROTOCOL FOR OPERATIVE MANAGEMENT OF TRACHEOSTOMY IN INFANTS AND YOUNG CHILDREN

1. Perform oral tracheal intubation and provide adequate ventilation. If a baby is alive, even though quite cyanotic and with an obstructed airway, an adequate orifice is available for insertion of an endotracheal tube (even if it is a very small one) with which to ventilate and temporarily oxygenate the baby. Even in the presence of inflammatory processes such as epiglottitis, the airway can be secured and an appropriately sized endotracheal tube placed by a skilled technician. Insertion of an endotracheal tube immediately converts a life-threatening, emergency situation into an urgent yet controlled operative procedure and avoids many of the complications formerly associated with emergency-hurried tracheostomy.

2. The baby should be given light general anesthesia in an operating room environment where there is appropriate light and instrumentation to conduct a major operative procedure. At least two individuals should be present for the operative procedure, and, preferably, a third should be on hand to act as a cir-

DON'T X   DO √

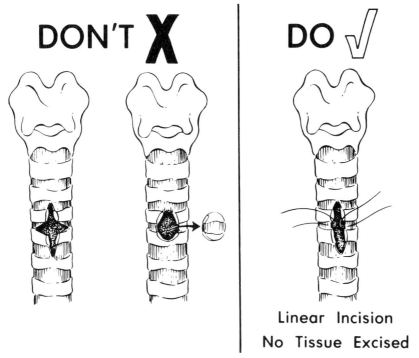

Linear Incision
No Tissue Excised

FIGURE 15–1. The two figures on the left are improper techniques for tracheostomy in children. On the right, note retraction sutures on the edge of the linear incision.

culator or scrub nurse. This sterile operative approach will decrease the possibility of contamination and subsequent infection with the inevitable fibrosis and granulation tissue. In addition, in small, fat babies, exposure in the neck can be difficult, thus making assistants necessary. A tracheostomy should be carried out only under ideal circumstances.

3. A transverse cervical skin incision, which is preferable for cosmetic reasons, is made, after which the cervical fascia is incised vertically in the midline. Because the thyroid isthmus can, under controlled conditions, be retracted out of the operative incision, it is rarely, if ever, necessary to divide the thyroid gland. Next, a vertical incision is made in the midline of the trachea, and one or two tracheal rings above and below the proposed site of the tracheostomy are incised. A mattress or figure-of-eight suture of 3-0 or 4-0 polypropylene or nonabsorbable Dacron suture is then placed through the tracheal wall on either side of the vertical incision. These sutures are kept long enough to come easily through the wound and be taped to the child's neck (Fig. 15–1). A sharp tracheal hook is placed in the most cephalad angle of the tracheostomy incision to steady the trachea and give counter traction; at the same time, an appropriately sized, snugly fitting plastic tracheostomy tube of proper length and configuration is inserted under direct vision while the anesthesiologist slowly removes the endotracheal tube. The skin is then loosely reapproximated, and the wings of the tracheostomy tube are sutured with permanent suture material to the lateral skin on either side of the opening. A sterile dressing is then applied and the child is nursed in an intensive care setting.

4. After a minimum of 48 hours (preferably 72 hours after the original tracheostomy tube is inserted), the tracheostomy tube may be changed; the child is either sedated or reassured by the nurse and/or parent during the exchange.

TABLE 15-1. Tracheostomy Tubes for Infants and Children

Characteristic	Shiley	Argyle
Construction material	Polyvinyl—more rigid but should be changed every 6–8 weeks because plastisizer leaks out	Silicone rubber—more limber, little tissue reaction, and material does not change
Available sizes	Neonatal: 00,0,1 Pediatric: 00,0,1,2,3,4	000,00,0,1,2,3,4,5
Ease of insertion	More rigid; has removeable obturator	More limber and more difficult to reinsert; no obturator
Connection to ventilator	15-mm adaptor rigidly a part of the tube; the tube may be dislodged when attached to ventilator tubing	15-mm adaptor is able to move and is less likely to dislodge the tube when movement occurs at the ventilator attachment
Ease of use	Is nonobtrusive and fits well into a child's neck	Elevated 15-mm adaptor is less likely to be obstructed by the large chin of a chubby child; can be removed to produce a flush tracheostomy tube

If, at any time during the first few postoperative days, the tracheostomy should become displaced, the nurse or physician attending the child can easily reinsert another tube by lifting up on the two mattress sutures located on either side of the tracheostomy opening; it is in this manner that the airway and entry site for the new tracheostomy tube are re-established. These temporary but vitally important mattress sutures are left in place for at least 1 week.

5. Extubation is attempted as soon as the primary disease process has abated and the airway has been carefully evaluated from above with an endoscope. If there appears to be no further endotracheal disease, only mild sedation and reassurance are necessary to remove the tracheostomy tube. Unless it has been in place for longer than 2 weeks, the tracheostomy opening will usually close spontaneously within 48 to 72 hours following removal of the tube.[2,4]

TABLE 15-2. Tracheostomy Tube Specifications

Tube Type	French Size	I.D.	O.D.	Length (mm)
Shiley				
Neonatal	00			
	0	3.4	5.0	32
	1	3.7	5.5	34
Pediatric	00	3.1	4.5	39
	0	3.4	5.0	40
	1	3.7	5.5	41
	2	4.1	6.0	42
	3	4.8	7.0	44
	4	5.5	8.0	46
Argyle (Dover)	000	2.5	4.0	32
	00	3.0	4.7	34
	0	3.5	5.4	36
	1	4.0	6.0	36
	2	4.5	6.6	40
	3	5.0	7.3	46
	4	5.5	7.8	50
	5	6.0	8.5	54
Silastic (Dow Corning)	1	3.0	5.5	35
	3	4.0	7.0	40
	4½	5.0	8.0	43
	6	7.0	10.0	46

Note: I.D. = inside diameter, O.D. = outside diameter.

6. Home management of a child with a tracheostomy tube is quite appropriate if the primary care giver is responsible and can be taught the basic principles of tracheostomy care. Visiting nurses are valuable as well for the reassurance and continuing education they provide outside of the hospital[3,14,18] (see Chapter 17).

Using this standard protocol, a very low incidence of complications is to be expected and rarely, if ever, will post-tracheostomy stenosis become a problem.[17]

Editor's note: We currently use Shiley (polyvinyl) or Argyle (silicone) tracheostomy tubes. Tables 15–1 and 15–2 are useful in deciding which tube to use.

REFERENCES

1. Abdereen E, Downes JJ: Artificial airways in children. Surg Clin North Am 54:1155, 1974
2. Dempster JH, Dykes EH, Brown WC, Raine PA: Tracheostomy in childhood. J R Coll Surg Edinb 31:359–363, 1986
3. Filler FA: Optimizing care for the infant with a tracheostomy. J Pediatr Surg 5:55–61, 1986
4. Filston HC, Johnson DG, Crumrine RS: Infant tracheostomy: A new look with a solution to the difficult cannulation problem. Am J Dis Child 132:1172–1176, 1978
5. Galvis AG: Custom made cuffed tracheostomy tubes for infants and small children (letter). Crit Care Med 14:261, 1986
6. Haller JA, Talbert JL: Clinical evaluation of a new Silastic tracheostomy tube. Ann Surg 171–915, 1970
7. Holinger PH, Brown WT, Maurizi DG: Tracheostomy in the newborn. Am J Surg 109:771, 1965
8. Lynn HB, VanHeerden JA: Tracheostomy in infants. Surg Clin North Am 53:945–952, 1986
9. McLaughlin J, Iserson KV: Emergency pediatric tracheostomy: A usable technique and model for instruction. Ann Emerg Med 15:463–465, 1986
10. Miller JD, Kapp JP: Complications of tracheostomies in neurosurgical patients. Surg Neurol 22:186–188, 1984
11. Othersen HB: Intubation injuries of the trachea in children. Ann surg 189:601, 1979
12. Price DG: Techniques of tracheostomy for intensive care unit patients. Anaesthesia 38:902–904, 1983
13. Rodgers BM, Rooks JJ, Talbert JL: Pediatric Tracheostomy: Long-term evaluation. J Pediatr Surg 19:258–263, 1979
14. Singer LT, Wood R, Lambert S: Developmental follow-up of long-term infant tracheostomy: A preliminary report. J Dev Behav Pediatr 6:132–136, 1985
15. Tepas JJ: Tracheostomy in infants and children. Ear Nose Throat J 62:484–488, 1983
16. Tepas JJ, Heroy JH, Shermeta DW, Haller JA Jr: Tracheostomy in neonates and small infants: Problems and pitfalls. Surgery 89:635–639, 1981
17. Wetmore RF, Handler SD, Potsic WP: Pediatric tracheostomy: Experience during the past decade. Ann Otol Rhinol Laryngol 91:628–632, 1982
18. Wills JM: Concerns and needs of mothers providing home care for children with tracheostomies. Matern Child Nurs J 12:89–107, 1983

chapter 16

The Use of Lasers in the Pediatric Airway

Lucinda A. Halstead, M.D.

The application of laser technology to airway disease was stimulated by the need for precise instrumentation in an endoscopic approach to the larynx and trachea. In the early 1970s, Drs. Strong and Jako produced an elegant micro-surgical instrument by coupling the carbon dioxide (CO_2) laser through a micro-manipulator to a standard operating microscope. This introduced virtually bloodless surgery of micrometer precision into the field of vocal cord surgery, where precision had formerly ranged from 2 mm at best to 20 mm if the vocal cord was inadvertently stripped. The precision of laser surgery stems from its ability to be coupled to micromanipulators and from the unique interaction of laser energy with tissue. This interaction limits thermal damage to 0.09 to 6 mm depending on the wavelength chosen, compared with 10 to 20 mm with cryo-surgery or electrocautery. The selection of a laser wavelength will depend on the type of tissue and the intent of the surgery (coagulation versus excision). Properly used, laser energy produces little edema and minimal scarring compared with cryotherapy and cautery. Improperly used, the intense energy emit-ted by lasers can produce severe scarring in the surgical field, severe injury to the patient, and potential injury to all the operating room personnel.

The CO_2 laser remains the principal laser for airway disorders in both adults and children owing to its unique ability to vaporize tissue with minimal sur-rounding thermal damage. The Neodinium-YAG (Nd-YAG) laser is reserved for highly vascular lesions owing to its intense thermal effect on large volumes of tissue. The potassium titanyl phosphate (KTP) laser has attracted attention owing to its small fiber delivery system. This laser has a greater ability to vapor-ize tissue than the Nd-YAG but can cause substantially more thermal damage to tissue than the CO_2 laser, severely limiting its application in the airway.

The purpose of this chapter is to highlight several airway lesions in which

POWER DENSITY

PD = power/spot size surface area

Varying surgical effects can be achieved by keeping the power and the duration of the beam constant and varying only the spot size.

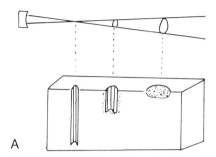

A

POWER DENSITY

PD = power/spot size surface area

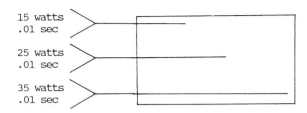

15 watts
.01 sec

25 watts
.01 sec

35 watts
.01 sec

The laser set at the highest power penetrates the deepest, when exposure time and spot size are constant.

B

FIGURE 16–1. *A,* Effect of varying the spot size on power density. As spot size increases, power density decreases. *B,* Effect of varying power output on power density.

laser energy has a unique advantage over cold knife, cryosurgery, or cautery excision and to provide a reference resource for laser surgery. Although surgical technique and instrumentation will be discussed, this chapter does not replace the "hands on," wavelength-specific workshops that the physician must attend to receive the in-depth training necessary to use each laser and to obtain hospital laser privileges. Information on courses for all wavelengths may be obtained through the American Society for Laser Medicine and Surgery, Inc.*

PRINCIPLES OF LASER SURGERY

Lasers are very intense sources of light. A moderately intense laser emits light more intense than that of the sun. LASER is an acronym for *Light Amplification by the Stimulated Emission of Radiation.* Although it is more correct to call lasers sources of electromagnetic radiation, it has become usual to refer to laser emissions as light since many lasers are in the near visible spectrum and can be focused, reflected, and refracted by lenses, mirrors, and prisms, as can visible light.

The key to successful laser surgery is understanding and controlling the interaction of each laser wavelength with tissue. The excellent, clinically oriented reviews of laser physics by Polanyi and of laser–soft tissue interaction by Shapshay and associates should be read by all laser surgeons.[10,11] The essential characteristics of the lasers most commonly used in the airway are summarized.

CARBON DIOXIDE LASER.   This 10,600-nanometer (nm) wavelength is strongly absorbed by water and all biologic tissue, with 90% of its absorption (i.e., thermal damage) occurring within 0.03 mm and 99% within 0.09 mm. Reflection and back scatter are negligible. The tissue absorbing the laser energy heats to $\approx 100°C$ and vaporizes. It is this property that allows the CO_2 laser to function as a "light scalpel" and cut with very little surrounding tissue damage. To maximize the properties of this laser, the principles of power density and radiant exposure as shown in Figures 16–1 and 16–2 must be understood. Oth-

*813 Second St., Suite 200, Wausau, WI 54401 (715) 845-9283.

RADIANT EXPOSURE

RE = power density x time

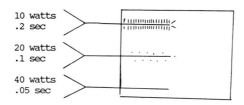

Radiant exposure is equal in each case.
Depth of penetration is equal in each case.
Thermal damage is greater as exposure time
increases.

FIGURE 16-2. Thermal effects of radiant exposure.

erwise, the ensuing thermal damage will yield results that are little better than electrocautery. The strong absorptive properties of the CO_2 laser make it a poor hemostatic agent for vessels larger than 0.5 mm in diameter.

NEODINIUM-YAG LASER. This 1060-nm laser is weakly absorbed in water. Its absorption is color dependent, with dark pigment and carbon particles causing strong absorption. The poor absorption in tissue causes strong scattering (thermal damage) in large volumes of tissue, with only 90% of the power being absorbed within 2 mm. These properties make the Nd-YAG laser excellent for vascular lesions, since even 1- to 2-mm vessels can be easily coagulated, but limit its effectiveness in most airway lesions where thermal damage leading to scarring and transmural injury must be minimized.

KTP LASER. This 532-nm laser has properties in between those of the CO_2 and Nd-YAG lasers. It is strongly absorbed by pigmented tissue and has variable absorption in whitish tissue. Its scattering (thermal damage) to tissue is intermediate to that of the CO_2 and Nd-YAG lasers, thus limiting its application in the airway.

EQUIPMENT AND SURGICAL SET UP

The technique and instruments used for laser laryngeal surgery are those of microscopic suspension direct laryngoscopy (Figs. 16–3 through 16–5). Once the lesion is visualized, the laryngoscope is stabilized or "suspended" by a holder, which allows the surgeon to use both hands. An excellent system is the Boston University Suspension System,* which applies a lifting force opposite the larynx, thus decreasing the potential for the upper teeth to be used as a fulcrum. It also maintains the larynx and trachea in straight alignment for use of the Venturi jet (Sanders) ventilation system. Pediatric laryngoscopes designed for laser laryngoscopy include the Jako and Dedo laryngoscopes (child size), the Healy-Jako pediatric subglottiscope, and the Ossoff neonatal subglottiscopes.† These scopes have a nonreflective finish for use with the laser and

---

*Pilling, Inc.

†All are available from Pilling, Inc., Fort Washington, PA.

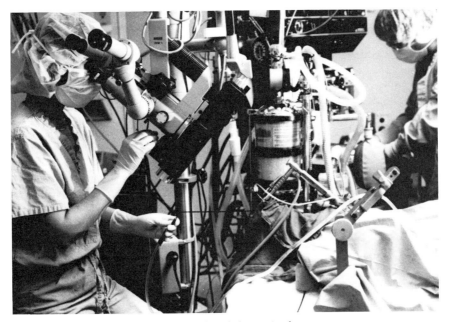

FIGURE 16-3. Carbon dioxide laser microlaryngoscopy.

have wide proximal apertures to allow for binocular vision through the operating microscope.

A variety of "mini-micro-" and "micro-" forceps, suctions, platforms, and scissors are made with a nonreflective or ebonized finish for use with the laser.* Nonreflective or ebonized finishes are imperative. Without them, reflective injury to the surgeon, endotracheal tube, and normal tissue will occur.

Laser energy can be delivered through bronchoscopes via fibers or micromanipulators. The physical properties of the CO_2 laser do not allow for fiber-

---

*Pilling, Inc.; Weck; Research Triangle Park, NC; Karl Storz, Endoscopy American, Inc., Culver City, CA.

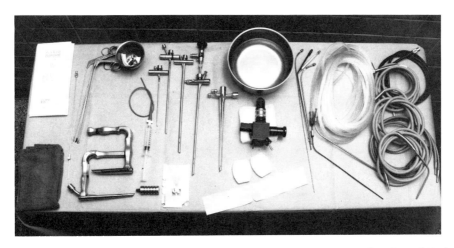

FIGURE 16-4. Laser microlaryngeal instruments (left to right): Venturi jet needle, Jako and Healy laryngoscopes, Boston University suspension laryngoscope handle extension, Storz bronchoscopes, laser bronchoscope, laser bronchoscopic coupler, microlaryngeal suctions.

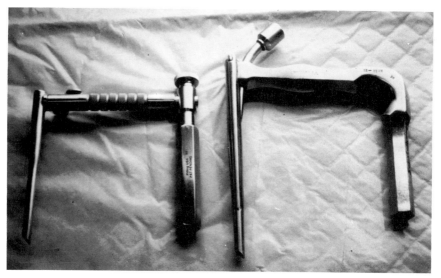

FIGURE 16–5. Healy pediatric subglottiscope and Ossoff neonatal subglottiscope.

optic transmission. The beam is coupled to a micromanipulator that reflects the beam down the bronchoscope.* The KTP and Nd-YAG lasers are delivered via quartz fibers. The small fiber of the KTP can be introduced through the sideport of the Storz bronchoscopes. The Nd-YAG requires a larger fiber and must be inserted directly into the bronchoscope tube.

Multiple CO_2 laser systems are available. In choosing a laser system, super-pulse capability and an "ultraspot" micromanipulator are desirable. Superpulse is a mode of delivering very high-intensity, short laser bursts with several milliseconds between each burst to allow for tissue cooling and decreased thermal damage. A very small spot or "ultraspot" micromanipulator differs from the standard micromanipulator accessory offered on most lasers in that it has a spot size of 0.3 mm at a 400-mm working length (the most common working length for microlaryngoscopy) versus 0.8 mm for standard micromanipulators. The advantages of a smaller spot size in a tiny airway are obvious. An excellent small spot micromanipulator is made by Heraeus LaserSonics.* This instrument has the additional advantage of a green fiberoptic aiming beam, which creates a virtual image on the surgical field and eliminates glare problems often encountered in small laryngoscopes with the helium-neon (HeNe) aiming beam furnished by the laser.

LASER SAFETY

Along with the advantages of lasers in airway surgery, the unique and potentially catastrophic complications must be considered. With proper precautions and meticulous attention to detail, laser surgery has been shown to present minimal risk to the patient, surgeon, and operating room personnel.[6] The participation in "hands-on" workshops that stress laser safety has been shown to dramatically decrease complications among surgeons who have not received

---

*Excellent systems are available from Pilling, Inc.; Karl Storz; and Wolf, Rosemont, IL.

adequate training during residency.[9] Some of the major and minor complications of laser surgery follow.

Complications Involving Operating Room Personnel

The surgeon and operating room personnel risk burn injuries from the laser beam by reflection of the beam off highly polished surfaces or misdirection of the laser beam if the surgeon fails to place the laser in the standby mode between applications. Mandatory when using lasers are nonreflective or ebonized instruments and a strict protocol by which the laser is placed on standby before the surgeon takes his or her eyes off the field or changes instruments. This prevents accidental misdirection and firing of the laser. Eye injury remains the greatest risk of laser surgery. Wavelength-specific glasses with side visors or goggles must be used by everyone in the room. Care must be taken that the optical coating is not scratched, or the eye will be at risk. Explosion of dropped gas cylinders and electrocution secondary to power cords crossing external cooling lines (KTP and Nd-YAG lasers) can also occur.

Anesthetic Complications

Excellent reviews of CO_2 and KTP anesthetic considerations by Ossoff and Freid and their colleagues should be read by all surgeons and anesthesiologists.[5,9] The recommendations for the Nd-YAG laser are similar to those of the KTP laser.

The most devastating complication of laser surgery is fire in the airway by ignition of either the endotracheal tube or carbonaceous particles in the airway. There is no completely safe endotracheal tube. Polyvinyl chloride tubes are highly flammable when struck by the CO_2 laser and should never be in the airway when the laser is in use. Completely clear polyvinyl chloride tubes without any labeling or radiopaque strips may be used with the KTP and Nd-YAG lasers with a 70% helium 30% oxygen mix. An ignition hazard exists if the concentrations of these gases fluctuate and airway fires have occurred with this system. The Norton metal endotracheal tubes are the safest. They will not ignite but may heat from repeated laser impacts, causing thermal damage to the larynx or trachea. The rigidity, lack of a cuff (important only for large children), and small internal diameter of these tubes can pose difficulties in ventilating the patient, making them unpopular with our anesthesiologists. The Rusch red rubber endotracheal tubes are used most frequently. These tubes will melt and eventually burn if subjected to high-energy CO_2 impacts, and the red color will preferentially absorb the KTP and Nd-YAG wavelengths. To prevent this, the tube must be wrapped with aluminum tape. The tape is usually wrapped circumferentially, with each turn overlapping the previous turn by one-half width. This results in a laser-resistant tube that is fairly flexible but also bulky, making it unusable in infant airways. The cuffs on the Rusch tubes should be inflated with methylene blue–colored saline and protected by moist neurosurgical cottonoids during the procedure. The blue saline will alert the surgeon to disruption of the cuff and help extinguish sparks. Many other "laser-retardant" tubes on the market are available in adult sizes only.

Venturi jet (Sanders) ventilation has the advantage of removing flammable substances from the airway and is our preferred method of ventilation. This

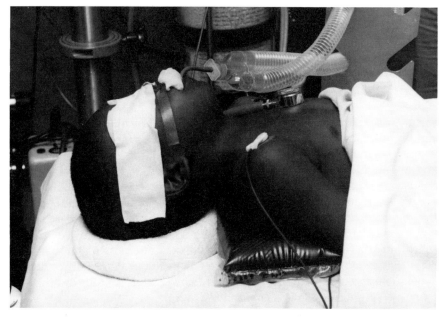

FIGURE 16–6. Patient prepared for CO_2 laser laryngoscopy with moistened eyepads and foil-wrapped Rusch endotracheal tube (foil not visible).

system delivers nitrous oxide and oxygen to the distal airway. Complications of this delivery system include hypoventilation from misalignment of the jet and pneumothorax secondary to air trapping behind an obstructing lesion.

The major hazard of laser bronchoscopy is ignition of anesthetic gases or carbonaceous particles. The use of helium is preferred as it does not support combustion as does nitrous oxide. Oxygen concentrations should be reduced to 30%. If higher concentrations are necessary for oxygenation, lower wattage should be used.

Patient Complications

Airway fires are the most catastrophic patient complication. Burn injuries to the eyes and face are the next most serious complication. Saline-moistened eyepads are suitable for use with the CO_2 laser (Fig. 16–6) but will not protect the eyes from the Nd-YAG and KTP lasers, since these wavelengths are not absorbed by water. Aluminum foil will reflect these beams. A prefabricated, adhesive aluminum foil eye guard with eyepads for corneal protection is commercially available.*

APPLICATIONS

Recurrent Respiratory Papillomas

Recurrent respiratory papillomas (RRPs) are benign lesions characterized by their frequent, occasionally relentless, recurrence after removal and their wide-

---

*DermaCare, Louisville, KY.

spread occurrence throughout the respiratory tract (nasal mucosa to lung parenchyma). The larynx is the most frequently involved organ. They arise from human papilloma virus, principally Types 6 and 11. Some evidence exists of an association of RRP in children and maternal condyloma. No form of treatment has proved successful in curing the disease.

RRPs are branching stalks of connective tissue containing multiple tiny capillaries and are covered by normal respiratory epithelium. Their great vascularity and affinity for the most constricted parts of the airway (larynx and subglottis) have posed significant problems to their removal. The CO_2 laser has become the modality of choice owing to its ability to bloodlessly vaporize the papillomas. The strong absorption of the CO_2 laser limits thermal damage to the tissue, resulting in minimal postoperative airway edema.

The goal of papilloma surgery is airway and voice preservation. Tracheostomy is to be avoided as it tends to cause dissemination of the papillomas to the distal trachea and bronchi. Owing to the recurrent nature of the disease and the multiple operations required for its control, scarring remains the major complication, with 32 to 36% of children having significant problems.[3,14] Anterior and posterior glottic webs are the most common sequelae. Scarring can be minimized using the following guidelines:

1. Vaporize papillomas to just above the level of the mucosa, leaving the submucosa uninjured.

2. Avoid circumferential removal of papillomas, thus decreasing the risk of stenoses.

3. Avoid removal of papillomas in the anterior and posterior commissures to prevent webbing.

4. Avoid lasering char or blood, which causes thermal damage.

5. Avoid "shoot thru" damage to the distal mucosa, which may predispose to distal seeding of the papillomas.

Acquired Subglottic Stenosis

Long-term intubation used in the management of neonates since 1965 is now the most common source of subglottic stenosis in infants and children. Whereas incidence rates as high as 20% were documented in the 1970s, current reports place acquired subglottic stenosis in infants between 4 and 8.5%.[2] These stenoses emanate from the loss of cartilage and soft tissue or the proliferation of dense granulation tissue followed by dense scar formation. Until the early 1970s, subglottic stenosis was managed primarily by tracheostomy and dilatation. The significant report by Fearon and Cotton in 1974 of a 24% mortality rate among infants and children managed in this manner has prompted a more aggressive approach to this problem.[4] Stenoses comprised of dense scar tissue have been successfully managed by CO_2 laser microlaryngoscopy, with avoidance of tracheostomy possible in many instances.[7,8] Twenty of 23 infants with severe subglottic stenosis treated at the Medical University of South Carolina have avoided tracheostomy or other open procedures in the past 2 years. The radial excision technique as described by Shapshay, in which portions of the subglottic cicatrice are vaporized, leaving mucosalized bridges between the lasered areas, was used on all patients (Fig. 16–7).[12] An average of two laser excisions have been needed. As inflammation from bacterial superinfection and gastric acid promote stenosis formation, these factors should be controlled in the perioperative period.

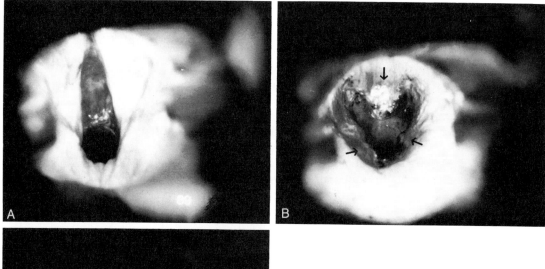

FIGURE 16–7. *A*, Subglottic stenosis, preoperative. *B*, Radial incisions with mucosalized bridges (arrows). *C*, Subglottic stenosis, 4 weeks postoperative.

Congenital Subglottic Hemangiomas

Subglottic hemangiomas are rare lesions associated with a significant degree of morbidity and mortality. They can be either capillary or cavernous in nature. Capillary hemangiomas most commonly occur in the posterolateral area of the subglottis in infants and young children. They can, however, be circumferential. These lesions produce airway obstruction but typically do not affect the voice unless the vocal cord is also involved. The carbon dioxide laser has been used to successfully vaporize capillary hemangiomas and produce a satisfactory airway. This can usually be accomplished in a single sitting and can often prevent tracheostomy.[13] Care should be taken to sequentially remove circumferential capillary hemangiomas and avoid injury to the underlying cartilage. Otherwise, circumferential subglottic stenosis will result. Cavernous hemangiomas can also occur in the subglottic area but are not confined to children. Owing to the size of the vessels (greater than 0.5 mm in diameter), the CO_2 laser is not effective in these lesions. Treatment with the noncontact and contact Nd-YAG laser has been effective owing to its ability to selectively coagulate and sclerose the large vascular lakes.

Webs and Synechia

Congenital and traumatic webs and synechia can be vaporized by the CO_2 laser. Thin gossamer webs are easily treated with either knife, scissors, or CO_2 laser.

In these cases, there is no particular advantage to the CO_2 laser. With thicker webs (several millimeters in thickness), the CO_2 laser is helpful in creating a precise, bloodless incision. Occasionally, the insertion of a keel may be necessary to prevent rewebbing.[1]

Intubation Granulomas and Redundant Supraglottic Tissue

Prolonged intubation can result in granuloma formation on the vocal processes of the true vocal cords, causing airway obstruction when extubation is attempted. The granulomas are fairly vascular and tend to recur if incompletely removed. Redundant supraglottic tissue, either congenital or resulting from repair of other laryngeal anomalies, can also prolapse into the airway, causing obstruction. Cup forceps removal of granulomas is imprecise, and remnants remaining on the cords predispose recurrence. As with granulomas, forceps and scissor excision of redundant supraglottic tissue is moderately bloody. Blood dripping into the airway predisposes children emerging from anesthesia to laryngospasm. The CO_2 laser can vaporize these lesions bloodlessly and precisely and thus decreases the chances of granuloma recurrence and laryngospasm.

Tracheal Stenosis and Granulation Tissue

Tracheal stenoses may result from cartilage loss or scar proliferation. Granulation tissue can form in the distal trachea or mainstem bronchi secondary to inflammation and irritation of endotracheal or tracheostomy tubes. The bronchoscopic CO_2 laser has been highly effective in excising both tracheal cicatrice and granulation tissue since it vaporizes the obstructing tissue with minimal surrounding thermal harm, as shown in the excellent study by Shapshay.[11] Nd-YAG and KTP lasers must be used with extreme caution owing to their increased scatter in tissue and risk of transmural injury. Regardless of the wavelength used, it is imperative that the laser beam be directed parallel to the tracheal or bronchial wall to avoid transmural injury, pneumothorax, and pneumomediastinum. With stenoses, utilization of a radial incision technique has been shown to reduce circumferential restenosis.[12] Ignition of char or anesthetic gases remains the major hazard of laser bronchoscopy. Utilization of a 30% oxygen 70% helium gas mixture (versus nitrous oxide) will decrease the risk of ignition. Ball valving obstruction of the mainstem bronchi by loose fragments of granulation tissue can produce severe hypoventilation, lobar collapse, or pneumothorax.

SUMMARY

When the use of any laser wavelength is considered, the fundamental question is whether it clearly confers an advantage over nonlaser surgery. The pathologic airway conditions described previously clearly benefit by the application of laser energy. The unique interaction of laser energy with tissue in these instances cannot be duplicated by any other surgical modality, making it reasonable to proceed in view of the severe potential complications associated with laser use. To select and use lasers wisely, the surgeon must be experienced in this form of surgery. Surgeons not receiving training in this technique in residency must attend "hands-on" laser courses and increase their facility with these techniques in the cadaver or animal laboratory prior to proceeding with operative cases. Once the principles of laser surgery are mastered, a very powerful and elegant instrument for airway surgery in children is added to the armamentarium of the surgeon.

REFERENCES

1. Cohen SR: Congenital glottic webs in children: A retrospective review of 51 patients. Ann Otol Rhinol Laryngol 94:1–16, 1985
2. Cotton RT, Myer CM: Contemporary surgical management of laryngeal stenosis in children. Am J Otolaryngol 5:360–368, 1984
3. Crockett DM, McCabe BF, Shive CJ: Complications of laser surgery for recurrent respiratory papillomas. Ann Otol Rhinol Laryngol 96:639–644, 1987
4. Fearon B, Cotton RT: Surgical correction of subglottic stenosis of the larynx in infants and children: Progress report. Ann Otol Rhinol Laryngol 83:428–431, 1974
5. Freid MP, Mallanpati SR, Caminear DS: Comparative analysis of the safety of endotracheal tubes with the KTP laser. Laryngoscope 99:748–751, 1989
6. Healy GS, Strong MS, Shapshay S, et al: Complications of CO_2 laser surgery of the aerodigestive tract: Experience of 4416 cases. Otolaryngol Head Neck Surg 92:13–16, 1984
7. Holinger LD: Treatment of severe subglottic stenosis without tracheotomy. Ann Otol Rhinol Laryngol 91:407–412, 1982
8. Koufman JA, Thompson JN, Kohut RI: Endoscopic management of subglottic stenosis with the CO_2 surgical laser. Otolaryngol Head Neck Surg 89:215–220, 1981
9. Ossoff RH: Laser safety in otolaryngology—head and neck surgery: Anesthetic and educational considerations for laryngeal surgery. Laryngoscope 99 (Suppl 48):1–26, 1989
10. Polanyi TG: Laser physics. Otolaryngol Clin North Am 16:753–774, 1983
11. Shapshay SM: Laser applications in the trachea and bronchi: A comparative study of the soft tissue effects using contact and noncontact delivery systems. Laryngoscope 97 (Suppl 41):1–26, 1987
12. Shapshay SM, Beamis JF, Hybels RL, Bohigian RK: Endoscopic treatment of subglottic and tracheal stenosis by radial incision an dilatation. Ann Otol Rhinol Laryngol 96:661–664, 1987
13. Wenig BL, Abramson AL: Congenital subglottic hemangiomas: A treatment update. Laryngoscope 98:190–192, 1988
14. Wetmore SJ, Key JM, Suen JY: Complications of laser surgery for laryngeal papillomatosis. Laryngoscope 95:798–801, 1985

chapter 17

A Practical Guide to Home Care of the Child with a Tracheostomy

Harriet L. Magrath, R.N., M.S.N.

The child with a tracheostomy requires specialized care not only in the hospital but at home. The progress he or she makes toward extubation is dependent not only upon the surgeon but also on the quality of care received at home. Lack of proper attention after hospital discharge may result in recurrent infections of the upper and lower respiratory tracts and the tracheostomy site. Such infections increase colonization of the respiratory tract and result in a delay in the surgical treatment of the airway problem owing to cancellations of scheduled procedures and treatment.

The success or failure of extubation is dependent upon the compliance of the family regarding the child's care and the quality of instruction given to the parents. Instruction for home care should be provided by one primary nurse, such as a case manager or clinical nurse specialist, and a respiratory therapist. This arrangement provides continuity and facilitates proper and organized assessment of the parents' progress.

Home care has changed dramatically over the past decade. No longer is the child sent home with a suction machine, catheters, and a vaporizer at the bedside. Standard home equipment now includes a battery-powered suction machine, which enables the child to be suctioned without access to electricity; humidity supplied by a tracheostomy collar and delivered by an air compressor and nebulizer; and a hand-held resuscitator bag. Parents are instructed in all aspects of care. They learn the routine business of suctioning and maintaining the tracheostomy site and the recognition and treatment of infections and emergency procedures, including the management of bleeding from the tracheostomy, respiratory distress, obstruction of the tube requiring replacement, power failure in the home, and equipment failure. Parents of children at risk for complications are instructed in cardiopulmonary resuscitation (CPR); cardiac and respiratory monitors for the home may also be provided.

Before their child has an operation, parents should be reassured that they will receive complete instruction and practice in home care of the tracheostomy and assistance with home equipment. Providing that the child is stable, actual instruction for home care is usually initiated the day after tracheostomy. It is commonly assumed that the family will need at least 1 day to become accustomed to their child's tracheostomy and the care provided by the nursing staff.

Instruction is usually given in three separate sessions and is provided jointly by nurses and respiratory therapists. It is important that the parents master the material in each session before advancing to the next one. Written material and model demonstration are used in addition to actual bedside care.

PART I: ROUTINE CARE AT HOME

Instruction should begin with a thorough assessment of the parents' level of knowledge concerning the tracheostomy. They should be reassured that they will become more comfortable with the tracheostomy as they become more knowledgeable about its care.

The child's condition should be explained in layman's terms to facilitate parental understanding and lessen the intimidation parents may feel when confronted with a seriously ill child. The term "narrow throat," for instance, can be used instead of subglottic stenosis. Actual tracheostomy tubes and models of the airway are used to enhance parental understanding. A tube of the identical size and type as that placed in the child is ideal for demonstration. Parents should examine the tube to assess its flexibility, lumen, and length. The use of a model will aide in explanations of both the basic anatomy and physiology of the upper airway, trachea, bronchi, and lungs and the placement of the tracheostomy and its purpose. A basic understanding of the physiology of breathing and the manner in which the tracheostomy provides an open airway for the child is demonstrated with emphasis on the maintenance of adequate levels of oxygen in the blood stream.

Suctioning

Suctioning technique is usually taught by the respiratory therapist. Many parents are unaware that the lungs normally produce secretions. They should be told that these secretions are produced to clean and filter the air the child breathes and that the tracheostomy now blocks their normal exit route. They should also understand that, for this reason, the child will often require assistance in clearing these secretions. If the child is not suctioned, secretions will often accumulate in the lungs and thicken, thereby promoting an environment suitable for infections or mucous plugs.

Parents are taught to suction their child whenever (1) secretions are heard bubbling within the tracheostomy or (2) the child exhibits signs of respiratory distress. When suctioning, parents should use sterile technique, either the one-

or two-glove method. The former is often easier for parents to comprehend since there is less confusion over the "clean" and the "dirty" hand. The procedure for suctioning is as follows:

1. Give the child four or five "breaths" with the breathing bag, using the ungloved hand.

2. Put a few drops of the saline solution, which helps to thin the secretions, into the tracheostomy tube using the ungloved hand.

3. With the ungloved hand, use the breathing bag to push both air and the saline into the tracheostomy.

4. With the gloved hand, carefully insert the catheter 2 to 3 inches into the tracheostomy tube or until the child begins to cough.

5. Cover the suction port with the thumb of the ungloved hand. In so doing, secretions will be sucked out of the tracheostomy tube. Take care not to suction more than 6 to 8 seconds at a time because the child cannot get air while being suctioned. Remove the catheter.

6. Give the child four or five "breaths" with the breathing bag to help replace the air that has been sucked out.

7. Allow the child to rest for 1 minute and listen for more bubbling. If he or she continues to bubble, the procedure may be repeated until the tracheostomy is clear.

Cleaning the Tracheostomy Site

The tracheostomy skin site should be cleaned at home with a cotton-tipped swab soaked in hydrogen peroxide and then another cotton-tipped swab soaked in water. This method, which uses less peroxide than is required in the mixing and use of a one-half strength solution, works best for home care. The one-half strength solution is undesirable for home use because it denatures rapidly and should not be kept for more than 1 day. If full-strength peroxide is used, it is important that it be cleaned from the skin with water to prevent dryness and irritation.

If granulation tissue develops at the site, parents must be aware of the need to have it removed by cauterization with silver nitrate. After they have been instructed in cauterization, they can then treat any recurrent granulations.

The tracheostomy site is usually cleaned and its tie changed daily. A tracheostomy tie should be changed in the following manner:

1. Cut a fresh piece of tracheostomy tape long enough to go around the child's neck two and one-half times.

2. Carefully insert the new tape over the old one, as if the old tape were not there. Then secure with a knot snugly on the side of the neck. Never cut the old tie until the new one is secured.

3. With the new tie firmly in position, cut and remove the old tie.

The tie change should first be demonstrated on a model and then attempted on the child. Note that a double loop around the neck is used and that a square knot, as opposed to a bow, is tied on the side of the neck; a bow might accidentally be untied by the child or a friend, allowing the tracheostomy to subsequently become dislodged. Also, if the knot is tied at the side of the neck rather than in the back, there is less chance of it being mistaken for clothing or a bib and being accidentally untied.

Humidity

An air compressor equipped with a nebulizer, tubing, and an infant or pediatric tracheostomy collar is used to provide humidified air to the tracheostomy. A vaporizer or humidifier is simply unable to provide particles of water small enough to reach the lower respiratory tract. Secretions unexposed to humidity become thicker and more difficult to suction and may result in a mucous plug, which can obstruct the tracheostomy. The thicker secretions may also predispose the child to lower respiratory tract infections.

The length of time a child needs daily exposure to humidity varies. Some children are able to attend school without humidity; others are not. As long as the secretions are thin, the child may be allowed, without humidity, to play, eat, dress, and so on. If the child is going to be traveling, e.g., to and from the hospital, he or she may be off humidity for the trip as long as there is frequent suctioning, using saline to keep the secretions thin. The sleeping child should receive constant humidity; it will keep the secretions thin and loose, enabling him or her to bring them up easily.

Chest Percussion and Postural Drainage

Although chest percussion and postural drainage are not part of routine tracheostomy care, teaching can begin at the first session. Chest physiotherapy (CPT) is usually taught by the respiratory therapist, and a chart depicting the various positions for the procedure is given to the parents for reinforcement. Note that a child should always be suctioned after CPT and that the procedure should not be performed immediately after a child has eaten or vomiting may be induced.

PART II: INFECTIONS

The second session of instruction on tracheostomy care is usually held on the child's 2nd or 3rd postoperative day. At that time, the material presented during the first session is reviewed with the parents. They should be able to state the purpose of the tracheostomy; understand the basic anatomy and physiology of the trachea, bronchi, and lungs; and provide their child with routine care at home. Home care, in this instance, consists of suctioning the tracheostomy whenever needed, providing care to the tracheostomy site once a day, and supplying humidity to the tracheostomy at night and as needed during the day to prevent thick secretions. Tracheostomy site care is then performed by the parents, either on the child or the model, and positive reinforcement is given.

The new material covered in the second session concerns infection. The parents are taught to recognize and treat tracheostomy site infections and upper and lower respiratory tract infections. They are also taught to treat erythema and drainage at the tracheostomy site by increasing the frequency of tracheostomy site care to three times per day for 3 days. In the event of a persistent infection, they are instructed to apply an antibiotic ointment such as Neosporin or Bacitracin to the site after cleaning.

Routine care at home is altered slightly in the event of an upper respiratory tract infection, since an effort must be made to prevent the infection from progressing to the lower respiratory tract. To promote thinner, looser secretions and good pulmonary toilet, parents are instructed to provide prolonged periods of humidification to the tracheostomy. As a result, more cleaning around the tracheostomy site may be required owing to the increase in the child's secretions.

Parents are taught to differentiate between a lower respiratory tract infection—in layman's terms, a "chest cold"—and an upper respiratory tract infection by noting a change in the color of the child's secretions (to yellow or green) and the onset of fever. If infection advances to the lower respiratory tract, the child's primary physician should be notified and a culture (with antibiotic sensitivity requested) obtained to determine if the patient should receive antibiotic therapy. If the child will be cared for at home, the following regimen should be followed until the infection has cleared:

1. CPT every 4 hours.
2. Suction after CPT and as needed.
3. Tracheostomy site care twice a day and as needed.
4. Humidity to the tracheostomy at all times.

PART III: EMERGENCY CARE AT HOME

In the third session, parents are instructed in the management of any emergency that may arise at home. The list is lengthy and includes (1) bleeding from the tracheostomy due to irritation, (2) bleeding from the tracheostomy due to erosion into a blood vessel, (3) respiratory distress, (4) mucous plugging of the tracheostomy, (5) changing of the tracheostomy tube, (6) power failure in the home, and (7) equipment failure in the home.

Bleeding from the Tracheostomy

It is imperative that parents be able to differentiate between bleeding from the tracheostomy due to irritation and that due to erosion into a blood vessel. They are instructed that any slight bleeding (less than 1 teaspoon of blood) is probably due to irritation of the tracheal lumen and is not abnormal. Treatment includes the regular use of saline during suctioning to lubricate the catheter and decrease irritation and increased humidity to the tracheostomy until the irritation has resolved. It is important to note that the air is less humid during cold weather. Consequently, a decrease in atmospheric temperature may promote drying of the tracheal mucosa and result in occasional bleeding.

Erosion of the tracheostomy tube into a blood vessel will produce excessive bleeding. If this occurs, parents should call on emergency services and alternate suctioning and ventilating the child until emergency personnel arrive for transportation to the hospital. In a critical situation such as this one, parents may abandon strict sterile technique and use "clean" technique for suctioning; in other words, they may suction the child with a catheter and gloves that are clean as opposed to sterile.

Respiratory Distress

Parents are taught to recognize the signs and symptoms of respiratory distress in a child with a tracheostomy. The treatment for this type of emergency consists of suctioning, using clean technique with the instillation of saline, and ventilation with the resuscitator bag. If, following this procedure, the distress is not soon alleviated or if insertion of the catheter for suctioning is impossible, the tube is probably obstructed with a mucous plug. Confronted with this situation, parents should change the tracheostomy tube.

Parents are actually required to change their child's tracheostomy tube while still in the hospital before he or she can be discharged to home care. For this reason, the child is usually hospitalized for a minimum of 7 postoperative days; the interim week allows for maturation of the tracheal stoma and removal of the stay sutures. Parents should practice changing the tube on a model before actually changing the tube on their child. Trial attempts on the model demonstrate the need for curving the tube during placement so as not to traumatize the posterior wall of the trachea during insertion. After they have practiced on the model, parents can observe while the physician removes the tracheostomy tube from their child and inserts a new one. Parents can then remove their child's new tube and reinsert it themselves.

The family of a child with a tracheostomy should receive at least two extra tracheostomy tubes, one the same size and type as that in place and one a size smaller in case the stoma closes and will not accept the original tube. If the child has a soft silicone tube, an extra tube with an obturator may be needed, since the silicone tube may not be firm enough for reinsertion. *These extra tubes should be kept with the child at ALL times.* The extra identical tube should be prepared for use. The tie should be inserted into one side of the tube and a pair of scissors should be taped to the package so that they will be readily accessible for cutting the tracheostomy tie in the event of an emergency tube change. The extra identical tube should also be taped onto the wall in the hall of the child's home; this is one of the few places where there is little chance of it being misplaced.

In addition to an extra tracheostomy tube, emergency phone numbers and specific directions to the home should be taped up on the wall as well; these should be near the telephone where they are readily accessible. The primary caregiving parent is usually needed to care for the child during an emergency; another relative, perhaps one unfamiliar with the quickest route to the home, or a neighbor, possibly one ignorant of the child's condition, will be the person who notifies emergency-care personnel.

Power Failure in the Home

Parents should be reassured that it is not necessary to have electrical power to care for the child with a tracheostomy. In the event of a power outage, the child's suction machine will continue to function, drawing power from its intrinsic battery pack. Also, humidity can be provided to the tracheostomy by the instillation of saline into the tracheostomy, after which the child should be suctioned.

If a power outage does occur, it is of primary importance that parents remain calm. If they panic, they will communicate their tension to the child, who will become upset and, in all likelihood, require more suctioning. Parents must remember that, even during an electrical outage, the telephone usually works. They may call a friend or relative who lives in another section of town where they may take their child until power is restored. A parent who has prepared properly for emergencies will have notified the electrical company of the child's condition upon arrival home from the hospital. The electrical company will then be aware of the presence in the home of a child who requires medical care and who is maintained with medical equipment powered by electricity. The home will then be put on the company's list for priority repair of any electrical problems.

Equipment Failure in the Home

Equipment failure should not pose a serious problem. As previously stated, it is not usually necessary to expose the tracheostomy to humidity on a continuous basis. Also, the home equipment supplier is required to provide a 24-hour call number through which he or she may be notified of equipment malfunction or failure. Upon notification, he or she must replace the inoperative equipment within 1 hour. The child will probably need suctioning during the 1-hour lag time; a DeLee mucous trap can be used temporarily for this purpose until a new suction machine can be obtained.

HIGH-RISK PATIENTS

Infants, especially premature ones, who are under the age of 6 months and have a tracheostomy are generally considered to be high-risk patients owing to the small size of the trachea. These children are usually kept on apnea and cardiac monitors until the age of 6 months. Their parents are instructed in CPR.

If the child requires oxygen to the tracheostomy, the appropriate equipment can be obtained from the durable medical equipment provider. In addition to routine equipment, this child will need an oxygen concentrator powered by electricity for a FIO_2 of 35% or less, liquid O_2 for a FIO_2 of greater than 35%, and auxiliary O_2 tanks for use in the event of a power failure and/or during transport. The durable medical equipment representative should instruct the parents in the care, use, and maintenance of O_2 therapy and all other equipment.

HOME EQUIPMENT CHECK LIST

1. Suction machine with DC battery pack
2. Air compressor with nebulizer, tubing, and tracheostomy collars
3. Suction catheters
4. Self-inflating resuscitator bag (specify infant or pediatric)
5. Hydrogen peroxide
6. Twill tape for tracheostomy tie
7. Scissors (two pairs)
8. Extra tracheostomy tubes (one identical trach tube and one a size smaller)
9. Cotton-tipped applicators
10. Saline, single-use vials
11. DeLee mucous traps (2)

TRANSITION FROM THE HOSPITAL TO THE HOME

The stress of transition from the hospital to home care is greatly lessened by the assistance of more than one family member in the care of the child. Provisions should be made for two people to be instructed in home care of the child with a tracheostomy. If the primary caretaker were to become ill, the child would require attention by another caretaker within the home. Responsibility must be shared if the child is to receive adequate care.

Both caretakers should not stay in the hospital the night before the child's discharge. One caretaker should be designated to provide care at home the first night following discharge while the other caretaker sleeps. It is not necessary for the caretaker to remain awake with the child throughout the night, but, typically, the stress level is so high the first night home that the parent gets little sleep regardless of the child's condition. The child may sleep either in his or her own room or in the parents' room, if preferred. Usually, after a few days, the caretaker can properly assess whether the child is able to sleep alone. A portable intercom may be placed in the child's room if the parent is uneasy about allowing the child to sleep alone.

Children with tracheostomies are allowed to bathe and shower normally. If water is accidentally splashed into the tracheostomy, the child will either cough it out or the water may be suctioned out.

If heavy dust or pollen is in the air or if grass is being cut, it is recommended that the child with a tracheostomy remain inside the house until the air is clear.

The child with a tracheostomy should return to normal activities, albeit under observation, as soon as possible. A suction machine, catheters, saline, and an extra tracheostomy tube should accompany him or her for care outside of the home. Assistants in the school system should be instructed in the care of the child while he or she is in school. Babysitters should also be trained in the care of the tracheostomy; informed babysitters will afford the parents some much-needed time to themselves away from home. Home life will adapt to the care of the child and the tracheostomy, and the child will be healthier and happier at home.

The following is a reprint of the instruction booklet given to families upon discharge:

Home Care of the Child With a Tracheostomy*

H. L. MAGRATH, R.N., M.S.N.

SECTION I: ROUTINE CARE AT HOME

A tracheostomy, often called a trach, is an incision into the windpipe or trachea. A tracheostomy tube is placed through the incision and into the trachea below the voice box. The purpose of a trach is to produce a good breathing passage. It is usually done to help a child breathe when there is a blockage in the trachea. The trach is placed below the blockage so that the child can breathe easily through the trach tube.

Below the tracheostomy tube, the trachea divides into two tubes called bronchi, each of which leads into a different side of the lungs. The bronchi divide into smaller and smaller tubes in the lungs until they eventually come in contact with tiny blood vessels. The "new" air which we breathe in goes into the tiny blood vessels; the "old" air which we breathe out comes out of the tiny blood vessels. The "new" air provides oxygen to the whole body—including the heart and brain.

The lungs produce secretions which clean both the lungs themselves and the

---

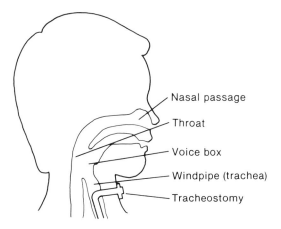

air within them. The secretions flow up out of the lungs through the trachea and are normally swallowed without the person realizing it. A trach prevents these secretions from being swallowed; as a result, secretions must come out of the trach tube. Some children with trachs can cough out all their secretions; many children, however, need help clearing their secretions. **If all of the child's secretions are not cleared, an infection may result or the secretions may thicken and actually block the trach tube. Complete blockage of the trach tube would prevent the child from breathing. Problems such as these are prevented with proper suctioning of secretions.**

How to Suction

A trach must be suctioned when: 1) secretions are heard bubbling in the trach and 2) the child shows signs of having trouble breathing. A tube called a catheter, which is attached to a special vacuum machine, is used to pull or suck the secretions out of the trach.

Be sure to wash your hands before working with your child's trach. To begin the suctioning process, you must first open the catheter and the glove package. The glove is worn on the hand holding the catheter in order to keep the catheter very clean so that no germs get in the trach. The outside of the glove must be kept very clean for this same reason. The wrist portion of the glove is folded up so that you can hold it to put the glove on your hand. Use the gloved hand to remove the catheter from its package and attach it to the suction machine tubing.

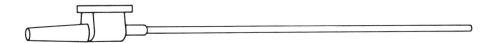

The suctioning process itself:
1. Give your child 4 or 5 "breaths" using the breathing bag to push air into the trach.
2. Using the ungloved hand, put a few drops of the salt water (saline) solution into the trach.
3. Using the ungloved hand, give your child 4 to 5 "breaths" with the breathing bag.

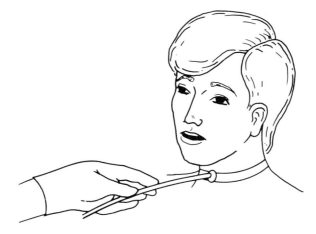

4. Using the gloved hand, carefully insert the catheter 2–3 inches into the trach.
5. Cover the suction port with the thumb of the ungloved hand. By doing so, secretions will then be sucked out of the trach tube. **Take care not to suction for more than 6–8 seconds at a time because your child cannot get air while he is being suctioned.**
6. Give your child 4–5 "breaths" with the breathing bag to help replace the air that has been sucked out.
7. Let your child rest for a minute while you listen for more bubbling. If he continues to bubble, the entire procedure should be repeated until the trach is clear.

Cleaning the Trach Site

The trach site is the place where the trach tube is inserted through the child's skin and into his neck. This area should be cleaned and all crust removed with a cotton-tipped swab which has been dipped in hydrogen peroxide. After cleaning, the peroxide should be wiped from the skin with a cotton-tipped swab dipped in water. In order to prevent a skin infection, the trach site should be cleaned daily and whenever the area seems dirty. The trach tie which goes around the child's neck and holds the trach in place should also be changed daily as well as whenever it seems dirty.

In order to change the trach tie:
1. Cut a fresh piece of trach tie long enough to go around the child's neck 2½ times.
2. Carefully insert the new tie over the old tie (as if the old tie were not there) and tie a snug knot on the side of the neck. *Never* **cut the old tie until the new one is secured.**
3. With the new tie knotted and firmly in place, remove the old tie.

Humidity

A child with a trach needs a machine called an air compressor that is equipped with a nebulizer to provide warm, moist air to his trach. Air is normally warmed and moistened in the nose and throat before it gets to the lungs. The child with a trach needs humidity to moisten the air that he breathes. Without exposure to humidity, a child's secretions will become thicker and more difficult to suction. Thick, dry secretions could block his trach and stop him from breathing.

Humidity should be used: at night, whenever the child is in one place for 30 minutes or more, and whenever the child's secretions look thicker than normal. The daily length of time a child needs humidity varies according to the child. Some children, for instance, are able to attend school without humidity. As long as the child's secretions are thin, he may be without humidity for an undetermined period of time for activities such as playing, eating, and dressing. If the child is planning to travel for a while, such as to the hospital or to the home of relatives, he may be without humidity for the needed period of time as long as he is suctioned frequently, using saline to keep his secretions thin. A child with a tracheostomy should drink plenty of liquids when he is off humidity for any significant length of time.

Review: Routine Care at Home
1. Suction the tracheostomy whenever needed.
2. Clean the tracheostomy site and change the trach tie every day.
3. Give the child humidity at night and as needed during the day.

Chest Treatments

Chest treatments (called CPT or chest percussion and postural drainage treatments) should be given to your child whenever he develops a chest cold. You should begin learning how to give these treatments now. A chest treatment consists of using your cupped hand to clap your child's chest and back in different areas. The firm claps keep the child's secretions loose so that they may be coughed up and suctioned out easily. During the chest treatments, the child is placed in varying positions which will be explained to you by your respiratory therapist (specific body positions allow secretions to flow more easily out of a child's trach than others). **The child should *always* be suctioned after these treatments.** Because it may shake his stomach and cause him to vomit, chest treatments should not be done immediately after the child has eaten. Your respiratory therapist will discuss these treatments with you in greater depth than we have done here.

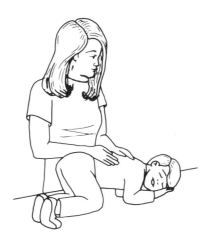

SECTION II: WHAT ABOUT INFECTIONS?

Tracheostomy Site Infections

The tracheostomy site may, at times, become infected. As a result, the skin around the trach will become red and irritated. When this occurs, the trach site should be cleaned three times a day for three days. After cleaning, care should be taken to wipe the peroxide from the site with a swab dipped in water. If, after three days, the redness remains or gets worse, an antibiotic ointment such as Neosporin or Bacitracin may be put on the area to help clear the infection. You should call your doctor if you have cleaned the trach site properly and put ointment on the area for 2 days, and the infection still has not cleared.

Head Colds

Ideally, your child should be kept away from anyone who has a cold or the flu. As we all know, however, children get colds, even with the best of care. If your child gets a head cold, he will react just as any other child would—he will have a runny nose and may have a mild fever. Your child may also have more secretions. When your child gets a head cold, you should do the following until the cold is gone to help prevent the cold from entering his chest:
1. Suction your child whenever needed.
2. Clean and care for the trach site once a day.
3. Use humidity longer than usual.
4. Offer your child plenty of liquids to drink.

Chest Colds

The child with a chest cold will have the same symptoms as the child with a head cold. The child with a chest cold, however, is more likely to have a fever and his secretions will probably change color and be either yellow or green.

You should call your doctor if you believe that your child has a chest cold. The doctor will check your child, may send some of his trach secretions for culture, and possibly prescribe an antibiotic for him. In order to determine in which part of your child's lungs the chest cold has settled, the doctor will listen to your child's chest and may get an x-ray of it. This information is important because you will need to know the area of the chest on which you should spend the most time during the chest treatments you will give your child at home.

Home care of the child with a chest cold should be done until the symptoms have stopped (usually about 2 weeks). To provide proper home care for your child with a chest cold, you should:
1. Perform chest treatments every 4 hours (even during the night). Remember, correct positioning during the treatments is especially important.
2. Suction your child after every chest treatment and whenever needed, always using saline.
3. Clean and care for the trach site once a day.
4. Provide humidity to the trach *at all times.*
5. Offer your child extra liquids to drink.

SECTION III: EMERGENCY CARE AT HOME

Bleeding from the Tracheostomy

Occasionally, suctioning or coughing may irritate your child's trachea and it may bleed slightly. You may see small amounts of blood when you suction his secretions or he may cough some blood up. If this occurs, be sure to use saline, which reduces irritation, whenever you suction your child. It may also help to keep your child on humidity for longer periods of time than usual. Remember, don't panic. Slight bleeding from the tracheostomy is not an emergency and the irritation usually goes away in a day or two.

If, however, your child is bleeding continuously or in large amounts (more than 1 teaspoon), you should call an ambulance immediately. While you wait for the ambulance to arrive, you should suction your child for 15 seconds and then "breathe" him with the breathing bag for 15 seconds. Repeat this routine over and over until the ambulance comes.

Respiratory Distress

If your child has respiratory distress or trouble breathing, it is easy to recognize and you can usually correct it. If your child is old enough, he will tell you that he is having trouble breathing and that he wants to be suctioned. If he is not old enough to speak or if he simply does not mention his distress, there are a number of signs you can look for:

1. You may notice a change in your child's color. If your child is having trouble breathing, he may become pale or turn a bluish color, especially around the lips and fingernails.
2. While breathing, your child may use his neck muscles or his chest wall may appear to sink in.
3. Your child may be restless and refuse to go to sleep.
4. You may just notice a general difficulty in breathing.

If your child is having trouble breathing, the immediate treatment is to suction him well. If a good suctioning does not help him breathe or if you are unable to get the catheter down his trach, a thick plug of mucous secretions may be blocking the trach tube. If this occurs, the tube must be changed.

Changing the Tracheostomy Tube

Your child's trach tube must be changed if it is blocked by mucous secretions or if your child accidentally pulls it out of place. Your doctor will show you the proper way to do this (as it is explained here). In order to change your child's trach tube, cut his trach tie and remove the plugged tube from his trach site. Next, carefully insert the new tube (with obturator in place), curving it downward into the trach site rather than pushing it straight back. Remove the obturator or guide. The new trach tie should then be tied around your child's neck. Your child should be able to breathe once the new tube is in place. If, however, he continues to have trouble, he may need some breaths with the breathing bag.

Before you leave the hospital, your nurse will give you extra trach tubes for emergency replacement. If your child has had his trach for less than 3 weeks, one tube will be the same size and type as the tube your child has in place when he leaves the hospital and the other will be one size smaller. If you need to change your child's trach tube at home, always try to replace the old tube with a new tube of the same size. Only if the tube of the same size will not fit should you insert the smaller one.

Both tubes, the one of the same size and the smaller tube, and a pair of scissors should be kept with your child at all times. Keep the obturator *inside* the trach tube and the ties inserted on one side. Always, after any trach tube change (especially if you have changed a tube which has been blocked and your child continues to have trouble breathing after the new tube has been inserted), your child should be checked by a doctor. You can take the child to an emergency room where a doctor will see him. Ask the doctor to give you another trach tube to use as an emergency replacement.

MY CHILD'S TRACH SIZE IS: _____.

Review: Respiratory Distress

1. Suction the trach.
2. If suctioning does not help, change the trach tube then suction the new trach.
3. Have the child checked by a doctor.

Power Failure

Storms may cause a power outage in the home. This is not an emergency, even if your child depends on suctioning to keep his airway clear. It is your job to remain calm so that your child does not get upset. Your suction machine should have a battery pack for power; as a result, you will not need electricity for suctioning. If the electricity in your house goes out and your child is on humidity, his trach collar should be removed since the air compressor and nebulizer do require electricity to work. Do not panic if this occurs—if you suction your child every 30 minutes, using saline each time, he will be safe without any extra humidity. If your child is on oxygen, he should be switched over to a portable tank.

When you arrive home from the hospital, you should immediately call your power company. Let them know that you have a child with a trach and that he requires electricity for long-term care. They will then put you on their priority list for immediate repair during power outages. You should also set up an alternate plan with someone who lives on another side of town. You can plan to take your child to this person's house if the electricity in your neighborhood is out for a long time. Remember, the telephone usually works, even if the electricity is out; you can call your friends across town to see if they have electricity and arrange to take your child to their home if their power is still on. It would be very unusual for the electricity to go out all over town.

Equipment Failure

If your suction machine breaks, your child may be suctioned by mouth with a DeLee mucous trap. Your nurse will show you how to do this. If the machine breaks or malfunctions, call the equipment company and they will bring you a new machine. They will have someone on call 24 hours a day to help you with any problems you may have with your suctioning equipment.

SECTION IV: HOMEWARD BOUND!

Before you go home, you should be able to do everything and understand everything we have covered in this booklet. If you need help with anything, please let us know! If you would like, we will have a nurse come out to your house to help you with any problems you have and assist you with your equipment and supplies. If you need us, call us!

The following emergency telephone numbers should be written clearly and taped onto the wall by your telephone. In a real emergency, you will be caring for your child; you will send someone else to call for help so it is very important that these emergency numbers are both easy to read and easy to find. It is also a good idea to write out detailed directions to your home and tape them, with the emergency telephone numbers, next to the phone. If the person who calls for help needs to tell an ambulance driver how to get to your house, he will have no trouble doing so with the directions already written out and by the telephone.

AMBULANCE _____

DIRECTIONS TO YOUR HOME _____

_____

_____

_____

_____

_____

_____

EQUIPMENT COMPANY _____

LOCAL DOCTOR _____

HOSPITAL/DOCTOR'S OFFICE (Daytime) _____

HOSPITAL/DOCTOR'S OFFICE 792-2123. Ask for the _____
(Nights & Weekends)

_____ on call

NURSING UNIT NUMBER

EQUIPMENT CHECK LIST

 1. Suction machine with battery pack
 2. Air compressor with nebulizer and tubing
 3. Suction catheters and gloves—Size _____ French
 4. Breathing bag
 5. Hydrogen peroxide
 6. Tracheostomy ties
 7. Scissors (2 pairs)
 8. Extra tracheostomy tubes _____—Size _____and _____
 9. Cotton-tipped applicators
10. Saline
11. DeLee mucous trap
12. Prescriptions—_____

Medications

Your doctor may prescribe medication for your child when he is discharged from the hospital. The most common medicine prescribed is Prednisone, which is a steroid. This is given to decrease swelling within the trachea after surgery. Prednisone can also cover up the signs and symptoms you would normally see when your child has an infection. So, if your child does not feel good or has a slight fever and is taking this medicine, you should call your local doctor and let him know what is going on. One other side effect of Prednisone involves your child's appetite. When on the medicine, your child will eat more, he may gain weight, and his cheeks may get puffy. Do not worry if this occurs; it will go away after he has finished taking the Prednisone. Along with the steroid, your doctor may prescribe an antibiotic for your child to take when he has left the hospital.

It is *very important* that your child take his medicine exactly the way the doctor told you that he should. If you cannot get the medicine or if there is any problem with it, please call your doctor here at the hospital.

After You're Home

SLEEPING ARRANGEMENTS

If your child sleeps in a crib, it may be placed in your room so that you can care for him more easily at night. If he has trouble breathing or needs suctioning, he will become restless or create a disturbance and you will hear him. If you prefer to sleep in separate rooms, you can purchase a portable intercom for your child's room or you can tie small bells to your baby's shoes or socks. Either way, you will hear your child, even though he is in another room, if he has trouble at night. Babies under the age of 6 months are usually placed on home apnea monitors. An older child, because he will wake up and come to you if he is having trouble and needs suctioning, can sleep in his own room with no problems.

ASSISTANCE

The responsibility of caring for your child must be shared—it is not a job for one person only. Another responsible adult (either a family member, neighbor, or friend) should be trained by you to help you care for your child when you are there and to take over for you when you are gone. If you become sick, for instance, someone else must be capable of caring for your child. The same is true for the many times you will need to get out of the house and take a break. You simply cannot do the job by yourself.

BATHING

Your child may take a bath or shower, just like he did before the surgery. Care, however, should be taken not to get water into the trach. If water does get into the trach, you will need to suction your child.

DUST

If heavy dust or pollen is in the air or if the grass is being cut, it would be best to keep your child inside the house where he can breathe easier. He may go outside with no problem once the air has cleared.

ACTIVITIES

Your child should return to normal activities—under supervision—as soon as possible after he has left the hospital. He may play with friends, go outside, or go to school—as long as someone is available to care for him. Remember, your child received a lot of attention from the staff, family, and friends while he was in the hospital. He will need for things to return to normal once he is home. He will need to return to his normal activities and he will need normal discipline from you. He is the same child he was before the surgery, only now he has a trach.

You should train your babysitter in the care of your child's trach. After you have done so, gradually leave your child with the babysitter for longer and longer periods of time as he/she becomes more capable and confident in the care of a child with a trach. Do not be afraid to leave your child in the hands of a responsible, trained adult. Remember, parents need some time to themselves too.

Your home life should adapt to the care of your child and his tracheostomy. He will be much healthier and happier at home than in a hospital.

part 5

Future
Directions

chapter 18

Future Directions

H. Biemann Othersen, Jr., M.D.

The primary aim for the future of surgery of the pediatric airway should be the development of techniques and tubes that will enable endotracheal intubation and tracheostomy to be performed and maintained without the tracheal injury that leads to scar and stenosis. Tracheostomy tubes have been improved over the years but they need further development. In adults low-pressure cuffs have been developed that allow intubation without the risk of cuff necrosis.

New laryngoscopes may permit the tracheas of small children to be intubated with less trauma. A magnifying instrument, the Bullard laryngoscope, is being used in small children. Lasers with small fiberoptic delivery systems, such as the KTP laser, should enable the excision of even small endobronchial strictures and lesions. Instead of merely awaiting such technical advances, however, current techniques for the establishment and maintenance of endotracheal and tracheostomy tubes should be constantly reviewed and reinforced. Just as hand washing, the value of which has been known for hundreds of years, needs constant emphasis, proper management of the pediatric airway requires daily reinforcement.

A final reminder:

1. Use tubes of the proper size; tubes must not be too large.

2. With endotracheal intubation, secure tubes and patients well to prevent the shearing forces that accompany movement of the tube or the head and neck.

3. Do not use cuffed tubes in children unless necessary.

4. Take meticulous care with tracheostomy tubes—clean the stoma and cauterize granulations.

5. Perform tracheostomy when the larynx and upper trachea are inflamed and edematous or when endotracheal intubation is prolonged.

6. Early repair of blunt or penetrating airway injuries gives the best results.

PRIMUM NON NOCERE
ABOVE ALL DO NO HARM

INDEX

Note: Page numbers in *italics* refer to illustrations; page numbers followed by t refer to tables.